DATE DUE

12-11-97	
MAY 11 1999	
GAYLORD	PRINTED IN U.S.A.

PATIENTS' PRIVACY

Patients' Privacy

An exploratory study of patients' perception
of their privacy in a German acute care hospital

IRMGARD L. BAUER

Avebury

Aldershot · Brookfield USA · Hong Kong · Singapore · Sydney

Published by
Avebury
Ashgate Publishing Ltd
Gower House
Croft Road
Aldershot
Hants GU11 3HR
England

Ashgate Publishing Company
Old Post Road
Brookfield
Vermont 05036
USA

RA
965.3
·B38
1994

British Library Cataloguing in Publication Data

Bauer, Irmgard L.
  Patients' Privacy: Exploratory Study of
  Patients' Perception of Their Privacy in
  a German Acute Care Hospital. -
  (Developments in Nursing & Health Care Series)
  I. Title   II. Series
  362.11

ISBN 1 85628 918 4

Library of Congress Cataloging-in-Publication Data

Bauer, Irmgard, 1954–
  Patients' Privacy : an exploratory study of patients' perception
of their privacy in a German acute care hospital / Irmgard L. Bauer.
    p. cm. -- (Developments in nursing and health care)
Includes bibliographical references.
ISBN 1-85628-918-4
  1. Hospital care-- Psychological aspects. 2. Privacy 3. Hospital
patients--Psychology. 4. Nurse and patient. I. Title II. Series
RA965.3.B39   1994
362.1'1'019--dc20   94-16735
                                                             CIP

Printed in Great Britain by Ipswich Book Co. Ltd., Ipswich, Suffolk

Contents

Tables and figures

Preface

There is an ongoing concern about the relationship of a patient's autonomy and self-determination, and the experience of hospitalization. Over the centuries Western medicine and subsequently nursing has been traditionally based on the biomedical model with its focus on physical aspects and the aim to cure the then depersonalized patients. During recent decades new philosophical currents have emerged, namely holism, which considers the individual as a unified whole of body and mind, and humanism with its emphasis on the quality of existence (uniqueness of an individual, autonomy, freedom of choice). Nursing as a discipline was particularly prone to influence from those currents because of the close encounter with individuals in exceptional circumstances, such as illness, who depended on help. The profession took on board issues like the patient's autonomy, self-determination, dignity and the importance of a patient's feelings and experience. The phenomenon of privacy as a basic human need had no place in the traditional model. The scarcity of reference to this issue in the literature reinforces this fact. However, if the slogans of 'holistic' and 'patient-centred' care are meant to be taken seriously, it is high time to examine this topic more closely.

The roots of many research projects lie in the researcher's current or remote biography (Lofland and Lofland, 1984). In addition, the researcher's own experience and preconceptions play an important part in the interpretation of the phenomena under study (Denzin, 1989). To illustrate the personal context in which this study was conducted I felt it necessary to outline my biography.

I started my training as a general nurse in Germany in the early 1970's, brought up with the very traditional view of human beings based on the biomedical model. 'Holistic' or 'patient-centred' care was not a part of the then nurses' vocabulary. What an innovation when suddenly the item 'consider patient's privacy' was added at the bottom of the list of many tasks to be performed for a 'patient suffering from xyz'! In practice it meant not to forget to use screens when the supervisors came to visit us students. For the rest of the time screens were neatly packed away in the most distant store on the ward. The other privacy-protecting measure was, as far as I remember, not to uncover the patient completely while giving a bedbath. 'Rolling up the sleeves' and 'getting the work done' had a much higher priority than considering the personal aspects of the target of all our efforts. While working as a nurse and ward sister I observed over the years that screens became more and more unpopular – not with the patients but with the nurses, because the frames were so bulky, heavy and inflexible. They finally disappeared from the scene. As a young nurse tutor I carefully added the 'consider patient's privacy'. I cannot outline what part tradition played in my mentioning it, but I trusted that the students were mature enough to know how to implement this task.

Being a person with a pronounced sense of privacy and displaying distinct territorial behaviour, it is rather worrying how much of one's personality can be suppressed when the role of a traditional nurse is played. Menzies' (1970) defence mechanisms come to mind.

Encounters with other cultures, however, uncovered my previous need for privacy and made me even more sensitive. I worked for several years in an Arab country, where public and private life was separated, the latter entirely taking place inside the homes. However, in contrast to common belief, within the boundaries of the home, there was not much privacy (as understood by the Westerner) left for the individual. Company is preferred rather than even temporary solitude. Personal belongings are accessible to anyone, only a small lockable chest is really considered private – until it needs to be opened… Personal matters even the most modern Westerner would not disclose easily to anyone are discussed openly. In this environment my own preference was in danger of constant violation. Only my immense interest in the country, people and culture as well as practical measures helped me to adapt and cope. Extensive travelling to other parts of the world confronted me with various difficult perceptions of privacy, and, although often putting on a brave face, many of these were quite intolerable for me.

After many years away, I had to collect data for a research project and came back to a German hospital setting. Detached from the routine, things suddenly appeared in a quite different light. Very often I found myself upset observing events that invaded a patient's privacy in one way or another. I often found myself thinking: if I were this patient I would complain, … I would not want this, … I would not accept that, and I wondered how the patient felt at that very moment.

Apologizing silently to all the patients I had cared for years ago, I decided to investigate how people perceived the privacy they experience when they are hospitalized, using interviews. To do that, it was necessary to set my own values aside (as far as possible) and examine the topic through the eyes of the patients. It was very clear from the outset that the topic had to be tackled using a phenomenological approach because gaining insight into the perception of those concerned was crucial. I had used this approach already in a former study on a different topic (Bauer, 1991).

Searching the literature, the first thing that startled me was that there was no precise definition of privacy. Also it was soon obvious that not just privacy but also related themes, important in the hospital context, had to be covered such as territoriality and personal space. The topic turned out to be so extensive that certain areas such as data protection in connection with information technology, confidentiality, ethical and legal aspects are not discussed here at all or are only briefly mentioned if appropriate. Very little research could be found that examined privacy and/or interrelated aspects from the patients' point of view, especially in acute care settings. No single study examining the German context, was found.

Chapter 1 of this book introduces the literature on privacy in general and on related themes. An attempt has been made to cover current knowledge on the topic in relation to patients and hospitals. In certain sections the work of few but established key authors appears. In Chapter 2 phenomenology and phenomenological methods are discussed and the choice of method is justified. A description of the development of the interview guide follows as well as an explanation of the method of analysis. The findings of the interviews are presented in Chapter 3. As well as the initial interviews, questionnaires based on the interviews were administered to a much larger sample of patients. Chapter 4 outlines the theoretical background of the measurement of attitudes and describes the development of the instrument. It also examines the analysis of the data which are offered in Chapter 5. In addition to interview and questionnaire, the patients were asked at both stages to rank privacy-invading events. Development of the ranking list and analysis are discussed in Chapter 6, the results in Chapter 7. A broad discussion of all findings follows in Chapter 8. Chapter 9 introduces a tentative formal theory of privacy and in Chapter 10 the study is evaluated.

1 Privacy and related areas

Privacy

Privacy and the problem of definition

It probably does not often happen that the opportunity arises to write about a topic which is largely ill-defined, at least by people who have to deal with it on scientific, legal, psychological, sociological or other grounds. Ordinary citizens, however, seem to have little difficulty with the concept of privacy, as Younger (1972) assumed.

Velecky (1978) recognized the difficulty of an exhaustive definition of privacy and agreed on this point with Younger. The latter named two reasons why the meaning of the word 'privacy' cannot be defined or circumscribed satisfactorily. The first reason is its emotive content, which is irrational in nature, the second is its dependence on standards, fashions and mores which change constantly. Younger, however, offered a list of suggested definitions but these are in fact definitions of the right to privacy. In his criticism of Younger's work, MacCormick (1974) highlighted the 'plain analytical and practical difference between defining x and defining a right to x whatever x may be' (p.76). Other examples of this distortion are Creighton's (1985) right of privacy as the 'right to be let alone or a right to be free from unwanted publicity, exposure or scrutiny' (p.15) and Ernst and Schwartz's (1962) right to be let alone.

Despite these difficulties, several authors have offered a concept of privacy. Cantrell (1978) and Gifford (1987) suggested the distinction of privacy concerning the person and his social interaction, and the privacy concerning information about this person ('solo-type privacy' and 'data-type privacy' by Cantrell). This interpretation seems to be justified because, although not specifically mentioned, most definitions cover both aspects. A selection of this kind of definition is presented here. Altman (1975) offered one of the probably most comprehensive definitions when he says, privacy is 'selective control of access to the self or to one's group' (p.18), which emphasizes the subject's decision to deny as well as to grant access. Robinson (1979) stated that privacy is often described as

> ...withdrawal, as controlled opening and closing of the self to others, and the freedom of choice regarding personal accessibility (p.20).

Other definitions are:

> A condition of an individual when he is free from interference by others in respect of his intimate personal interests
> (The Report on the Law of Privacy, New South Wales, 1973, cited in Ashenhurst, 1978).

> A person's feeling that others should be excluded from something which is of concern to him, and also a recognition that others have a right to do this (Bates, 1964).

Westin (1967), however, seemed to concentrate on the disclosure of data when he called privacy 'the claim of individuals, groups, or institutions to determine for themselves when, how, and to what extent information about them is communicated to others' (p.7). Warren and Brandeis (1890) applied the same to thoughts, sentiments and emotions. Velecky (1978) criticized this view as too narrow and preferred the concept of 'being alone'. On the other side it can be questioned if this definition is broad enough to include every aspect, especially when concepts of person-centred privacy or information-centred privacy are also difficult to define.

This brings us back to Gifford (1978) and his statement that 'any attempt to define privacy precisely risks excluding some important aspects of privacy, overly broad definitions risk meaninglessness' (p.199).

The subjective structure of privacy

Bates (1964) interpreted privacy as a self-related subjective experience. He compared the self with a house, its rooms representing different aspects of the self image. The access to these rooms by others is limited to different degrees. He also suggested three different ways in which a person's privacy is structured:

1 Privacy is differentiated into many content areas. 'People doubtless vary a good deal in the specific areas which have privacy meanings attached to them, and in the relative strength of these privacy feelings for a given area' (p.430).

2 Privacy is structured by the degree to which certain people are excluded from having knowledge about somebody.

3 Privacy is structured by situational contexts, for example professional privacy.

2

Bates' concept of privacy strongly represents a phenomenological perspective. This, he stated, is also the reason why the experienced world a person calls private doesn't alter within short time spans, because the self does not quickly undergo radical changes.

Degrees of privacy

In his often cited book *Privacy and Freedom* Westin (1967) defined four distinct states of individual privacy. The first state is called *solitude* and represents the popular notion of privacy. It describes the individual's separation from the group and his freedom from observation. Solitude is the most complete state of privacy an individual can achieve. However, the voluntary nature of solitude has to be emphasized in contrast to isolation which is forced upon a person (Ingham, 1978). The second state, *intimacy*, refers to the seclusion of pairs or small groups to achieve either maximally personal relationships or maximally efficient working conditions. Intimacy can result in relaxed relations or wearing hostilities (Freud, 1960); it is, however, necessary to meet the basic need of human contact. *Anonymity* is the state where the individual is in a public place and free from personal identification or surveillance. Another aspect of this state is the anonymous publication of ideas. The fourth state is the creation of psychological barriers and is called *reserve*. It is the chosen limitation of communication with others. These above mentioned states vary considerably but their common feature is the freedom of choice of disclosure or concealment which an individual or a group has. Even if there exists a breach of privacy, the individual's subjective feeling of privacy persists as long as he is unaware of the intrusion (Ingham, 1978), which links easily with the importance of the experience of the self discussed by Bates (1964). This view was also represented by McCloskey (1971), who distinguished between negative liberty and breach of privacy and argued that a person's privacy can be totally invaded without his knowledge and, therefore, without interfering in his freedom of thought or action.

Functions of privacy

The human being is said to be a social creature, yet he constantly seeks to achieve a state of privacy. If he is deprived of satisfying this need, serious disturbances can occur. Hence the question arises what the functions of privacy are. It is again Westin (1967) who offered four functions which are not entirely separate but overlap and constantly flow into one another:

1 *Personal autonomy*. This function refers to the belief in the uniqueness of the human being and his worth as an individual. The need not to be dominated by others is maintained through individuality. Some authors like Goffman (1959) described interpersonal relationships in terms of zones, circles or regions of privacy around the 'core self'. In this inner area are located all those secrets and

thoughts which are not normally shared with anyone. An intrusion into this inner zone would be the most serious threat to an individual's autonomy. Ingham (1978) claimed that feelings of personal autonomy are reinforced by the possession of space for oneself. The different degrees of disclosure correspond with the backstage behaviour described by Goffman (1959). This behaviour is not supposed to be presented to the public.

2 *Emotional release.* Normative behaviour does not allow extremes of emotions publicly. Privacy can provide relief from the tension created by playing multiple roles in society. 'Privacy operates as a kind of a buffer between social pressures upon the individual and his response to these...' (Bates, 1964:433). This also serves as a 'safety-valve' to relieve emotional pressure and, thirdly, allows nonconforming behaviour.

3 *Self-evaluation.* This function describes the process of digesting experiences and gaining some meaningful perspectives. 'After bruising contact with the world, privacy may be required within which self-esteem can be restored' (Bates, 1964:433). It also allows the opportunity to 'step back' and think creatively.

4 *Limited and protected communication.* This function serves firstly as an opportunity to share confidences only with certain trustworthy individuals where one can expect that no disclosure of the knowledge to unauthorized people would occur. It applies also to communication with certain groups, such as physicians, lawyers and so on on whom the client can depend on confidentiality. Secondly, it sets boundaries of mental distances in interpersonal relationships ranging from the most intimate to the most formal.

In contrast to Westin's framework, Altman's (1975, 1977) functions of privacy concentrate more on the ability of a person or a group to interact with others. He named (a) the management of social interaction, (b) the establishment of plans and strategies for interacting with others, and (c) development and maintenance of self-identity as the goals of privacy (1977:68) and stated,

>...privacy mechanisms define the limits and boundaries of the self. When the permeability of those boundaries is under the control of a person, a sense of individuality develops. But it is not the inclusion or exclusion of others that is vital to the self-definition; it is the ability to regulate contact when desired. If I can control what is me and not me, if I can define what is me and not me, and if I can observe the limits and scope of my control, then I have taken major steps toward understanding and defining what I am. Thus privacy mechanisms serve to help me define me. Furthermore, the peripheral functions toward which control is directed – regulation of interpersonal interaction and

4

self/other interface processes – ultimately serve the goal of self-identity (Altman, 1975:50).

Altman's model of privacy-regulation, which will be discussed later, is derived from these three functions.

Schwartz (1968) interpreted privacy as a highly institutionalized mode of withdrawal. He stressed the group-preserving function of privacy that makes life with at times unbearable persons easier and stated that 'members of a stable social structure feel that it is not endangered by the maintenance of interpreted boundaries' (p.742).

Theories of privacy

Selective control of access to self (Altman, 1975). According to Altman, privacy is a three-dimensional process consisting of (1) a boundary control process, where dynamic and dialectic interaction with others takes place, (2) an optimization process, where the individual reaches the desired state of privacy, i.e. not too much and not too little, and (3) a multi-mechanism process, because numerous ways of regulating privacy are available.

Multidimensional developmental theory (Laufer and Wolfe, 1977). Laufer and Wolfe expanded the above named concept of privacy and included the factors life cycle, culture and time. They demonstrated how the perception of privacy changes during the individual's life and under cultural differences.

Hierarchy of privacy needs (Sundstrom, Herbert and Brown, 1982). After studying privacy in offices, Sundstrom argued that privacy needs are organized in hierarchical fashion, i.e. on lower job levels other needs exist than on higher job levels. One can question if the personal needs of privacy can be determined and/or met by this assumed hierarchical need of privacy.

As these theories of privacy show, there seems to be no model that is comprehensive. On can argue that this is small wonder since there is also no comprehensive definition of privacy.

Variables influencing privacy

Different factors influence a person's perception of and need for privacy. Some of these aspects are discussed here briefly.

Personal and situational factors. Upbringing, personality and social interaction combine to influence the desired or the actually obtained privacy. An interesting aspect was developed by Ingham (1978). He highlighted power and friendship as two of the most important dimensions of interpersonal relationship influencing, therefore, privacy. When power dictates the relationship, information flows in only one direction, invasion of privacy occurs only in one direction. Institutions may serve as a good example (Goffman, 1961). In some role-relationships invasion of privacy on the basis of power is accepted, for example with policemen. If the relationship is based on friendship, information will be disclosed gradually on a voluntary basis. 'The target person is, of course, an important determinant of the degree of self-disclosure, as is the extent to which reciprocity occurs' (Ingham, 1978:54).

Culture. Studies of different cultures have enlarged the understanding of the importance of cultural values for the individual's behaviour. The question arose whether all cultures needed the same amount of privacy. At first sight it seems that different societies vary widely in the amount of privacy the individual actually has. Lee (1959) studied different cultures like the Tikopia in Polynesia or the Wintu in North America and demonstrated the variations of privacy maintaining behaviour. More about cultural aspects of privacy can be found in Roberts and Gregor (1971). Altman and Chemers (1980) examined privacy regulations in other cultures from different perspectives. One distinguishing feature was if the society appeared to have a lot or very little privacy. They described cultures with obviously limited accessibility through others, and, in contrast, societies which seem to have no privacy at all. The author herself spent several years in an Arab country representing the first type of culture and stayed briefly with the BaMbuti Pygmies in the Ituri Forest in Zaïre where to the Western observer private life seems to be equivalent to public life. Extensive studies have shown, however, that all cultures seem to have the same need of privacy, yet they have different methods of preserving it. By not knowing these differences we may embarrassingly fail to understand privacy regulations in other societies. Most of these studies were conducted among non-Western societies. Hall (1966) examined one aspect of privacy, personal space, also among Western cultures. His findings will be discussed in a later section. Answering the question if privacy is culturally universal or culturally specific, Altman (1977) drew the conclusion that it is on one hand 'a culturally universal process involving dynamic, dialectic, optimization features', and on the other hand 'a culturally specific process in terms of mechanisms used to regulate social interaction' (p.66).

Regulation of privacy
As the reported literature demonstrates, the concept of privacy is closely linked to the individual and his individual need of privacy. For Etzioni (1968) need means simply that 'the person can be denied a specified kind of experience only at the cost of an intra-personal tension' (p.871). A certain degree of privacy may, therefore, be too much for one subject and too little for another. There can be many forms of intrusion into one's privacy, be it physical intrusion into the personal space, unwanted publicity, disclosure of private information, grave or

6

subtle, going as far as for example reading a newspaper over one's shoulder (Young, 1978). Intrusion into privacy can happen accidentally but also on purpose, 'a calculated invasion of privacy that would ordinarily be regarded as a far from rare form of aggression' (Bates, 1964:432). There is, however, another form of invasion of privacy that is professionally justified because it is essential for the professional relationship. It applies to priests, lawyers, in the medical field to nurses, physicians, social workers and so on. The Codes of Conduct of these professions emphasize that

> …penetration of a person's privacy carries with it the obligation not to reveal what is learned in any way which further reduces that privacy and thus potentially threatens the individual (Bates, 1964:432).

The individual needs to control the amount and degree of invasions in his privacy and to seek a balance which is right for him. Either too much or too little can cause an imbalance which creates serious problems. Too little privacy can be caused by environmental, economic, political, social, cultural factors. This means that functions of privacy cannot be utilized and stress is likely to be experienced. Too much privacy can arise through social or physical conditions beyond the individual's control or through an individual's failure to adjust to a successful daily life. It can cause and reflect a reduced communication leading to the frustration of motives which can only be satisfied in interpersonal relations (Bates, 1964; Westin, 1967). The individual must, therefore, constantly seek an adjustment between the counteracting needs of solitude and companionship. To regulate this balance people use a variety of behavioural mechanisms. The most complex framework of privacy regulation was developed by Altman (1975, 1977). It will be described in the next section.

Dialectic model of privacy regulation
Altman's model of privacy regulation is based on his three-fold theory of boundary control, optimization and multi-mechanisms. He identified four behavioural mechanisms which are used by the individual either solely or in combination: (1) verbal behaviour, (2) nonverbal behaviour, (3) environmental behaviour and (4) cultural practices. They will be discussed here briefly.

Verbal behaviour. The content of verbal communication but also paralinguistic cues such as voice quality, pronunciation and so on convey the information whether the individual permits access or not.

Nonverbal behaviour. Determining personal space or/and body language are used to regulate desired privacy.

7

Environmental behaviour. Clothes are one way to define boundaries. Casual clothes allow approach easily, uniforms or formal outfits keep people more at a distance. Our physical environment can be arranged in a way that reflects our availability to others. Personal space, the invisible boundary around a person serves also as a regulation mechanism. This topic will be discussed in depth in another section of this chapter. Goffman (1961) demonstrated how in institutions residents are not able or are not allowed to utilize environmental privacy mechanisms by using institution clothes and by architectural manipulation of the environment.

Cultural practices. Practices based on cultural norms, rules, and customs are named as a fourth aspect of privacy regulation.

Privacy-Regulation Mechanism

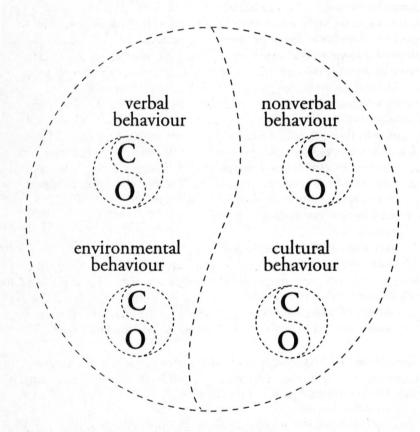

Figure 1.1   The dialectic model of privacy regulation
(after Altman and Chemers, 1980)

The large circle represents a person. Its boundaries are sometimes closed and sometimes open and 'permeable', demonstrated by the broken lines. The four above mentioned mechanisms are reflected in the four small circles, again in broken lines to show the opening/closing process. Each circle is divided into a closed (C) and an open (O) area, the changing accessibility is depicted on the basis of the concept of dialectics. The four mechanisms can vary in size depending on the immediate need of regulation and appropriateness.

Altman's model seems to cover all relevant regulation mechanisms. What should not be accepted without contradiction is the separation of cultural practices from the other behaviours. One can argue that cultural practices consist largely of verbal, nonverbal and environmental mechanisms and it seems to be more sensible to name culture as the all-embracing basis which influences the other forms of behaviour.

Research on privacy

Considering the emotive content of the issue it is small wonder that there has not been much research done on privacy. Up to now no comprehensive measure of privacy has been developed. Ingham (1978) listed some reasons why little research data can be found:

1 There is a logical problem in investigating a personal area that is by its nature closed to scrutiny. 'After all, in order to study privacy behaviour by field observation, the investigator is almost forced to violate the subject's privacy' (Gifford, 1987:201).

2 Data collection relies upon honesty. The researcher has to be sure that social desirability response bias does not threaten his results.

3 Ethical issues are another reason for either not conducting the research at all or not using confidential results. As protecting confidentiality might sometimes be problematic, a growing reluctance on the part of the public to participate in research can be observed (Fields, 1977). A number of authors have highlighted ethical problems connected with research. Only two examples are provided here:

> When the qualitative researcher delves into the private world and experiences of subjects, sometimes evoking strong emotional responses, and sometimes pursuing thoughts that might otherwise never be revealed, consideration of the common ethical issues may not be enough (Cowles, 1988:163).

> Ethics is a matter of principled sensitivity to the rights of others. Being ethical limits the choices we can make in the pursuit of truth. Ethics say that while truth is good, respect for human dignity is better, even if, in the extreme case, the respect for human dignity leaves one ignorant of human nature (Cavan, 1977:810).

4 The considerable influence of the behaviourist tradition on modern psychology and its quantitative research methods are not suitable for the investigation of taboos. One can, however, argue that this is no longer true as qualitative research methods became a well-established approach to investigating sensitive topics.
5 Linking with the previous aspect, privacy is in a sense a non-behaviour of a seemingly inactive non-directional nature and therefore not observable.

Territoriality

One of the issues related to privacy is the concept of territoriality. Derived from its application to animal behaviour human territoriality has been studied since the 1920s (Altman, 1975; Reid, 1976). Comparing the definitions of many authors (for example, Goffman, 1963; Lyman and Scott, 1967; Sundstrom and Altman, 1974), several common themes demonstrate the complexity of the issue:

- There is control and ownership of a place or object on a temporary or permanent basis.
- The place or object may be small or large.
- Ownership may be by a person or group.
- Territoriality can serve any of several functions, including social functions and physical functions.
- Territories are often personalized or marked.
- Defence may occur when territorial boundaries are violated.

(Altman and Chemers, 1980:121)

There exist several theories of territoriality, some based on the concept based on genetic heritage, others prefer learning as the determinant of behaviour, brain structure or conflicts. These theories, however, are controversial, speculative and mostly not research based (Gifford, 1987). Factors influencing territoriality are similar to those influencing privacy, namely personal factors (men occupy a larger space than women), social situation and cultural background.

As territorial events can be related to different aspects, Altman (1975) offers three distinct types of territories which relate in some way to the sociological classification of social groups.

Primary territories

Primary territories are owned and used exclusively by individuals or groups, are clearly identified as theirs by others, are controlled on a relatively permanent basis, and are central to the day-to-day lives of the occupants (p.112).

Examples are a person's bed, locker, bedroom, home, property, a nation's land. They are usually under the complete control of the owner(s) and lead to serious defensive actions in case of unwanted intrusions. It can be assumed that the inability to control primary territory (called personal territories by Goffman, 1961) in an appropriate way could lead to a deterioration of psychological well-being. The relation between control of primary territory and social behaviour was demonstrated by Altman and Haythorn (1967).

Secondary territories
They are less exclusive and less under the control of their occupants. Examples are the neighbourhood street, a social club, different areas in a town populated by different ethnic groups. They are available to the public, yet somehow under the control of their users. Goffman (1961) used the term 'group territories' but seemed to agree that those are situated between primary and public territories, i.e. they have elements of public access but are under a certain control by the users.

Public territories
Public territories like parks, bus seats, beaches, restaurant tables, shopping areas can be used by almost anybody on a temporary basis, provided that certain social rules are adhered to. Goffman (1971) described eight types of public territories (free territories), three are mentioned here. *Stalls* are public spaces available for temporary claims, like telephone boxes. *Turns* refer to places in a line, like at a supermarket checkout or a cinema, to get access to some kind of resource or place. *Use space* is the area around or in front of a person which is temporarily acknowledged as under their control, like the line of vision of a person who watches a painting in a museum.

Lyman and Scott's (1967) 'home' territories correspond to the secondary territories as do their 'interactional' territories that refer to any area where a social gathering may occur. Altman's primary territory is only partially replaced by the much narrower 'body' territory which includes the anatomical space of the body and the space occupied by it.

Functions of territorial behaviour
Two main reasons for human territoriality can be outlined: the management of personal identity, and the regulation of social systems (Altman and Chemers, 1980). The first function helps to illustrate the boundary between the person and others by personalizing a territory, for example through decoration. This demonstrates one's distinctiveness from others, puts a personal stamp on the place and allows the presentation of oneself to others. The second function regulates the 'social process, including control over various resources' (p.137) and allows to carry on with life's functions in a systematic way which is necessary for physical and psychological survival. The linkage between a func-

11

tioning social system and effective territoriality is demonstrated in several studies (Altman and Haythorn, 1967; Sundstrom and Altman, 1974).

Territorial behaviour and boundary regulations

To secure the above mentioned functions certain behaviour has to be employed. One way of doing this is to *mark* territorial boundaries (Goffman, 1971). Human beings use geographic indicators or artefacts and symbols. Walls, fences, hedges, nameplates are suitable means, but also in public places marking of temporarily occupied space occurs, such as for instance books on a library table or a coat protecting a reserved seat. The definition of a boundary is often evident through *occupancy and use* of a certain place. The simple presence of occupants prevents others from intruding and using the same space. Benches in a park which are already occupied by one person will only be used by a second when no other empty bench is available. An interesting point in this connection is that human territorial behaviour plays a role when architectural design is utilized for crime prevention (Merry, 1981). With justification, Sebba and Churchman (1983) pointed out that territorial behaviour is mostly considered in negative expressions like defence, warning, violation, intruding. Very rarely positive territorial behaviour like hospitality is mentioned.

Research in human territoriality

Relatively little research has been done on human territorial behaviour. Three major methodological approaches are used for studies of territoriality. Observation of behaviour in a natural setting provides rich data, used for example by Sundstrom and Altman (1974). Experimental studies exist as well. One must assume that territoriality needs some time to develop, therefore, subjects have to stay at least for several days in a laboratory (see Altman and Haythorn's study). Self-report methods such as questionnaires or interviews are a third research approach, used for example by Sebba and Churchman (1983).

Personal space

The idea of personal space deals with the boundary around the individual which is used to keep other individuals on a suitable distance, a 'body-buffer zone' (Horowitz, 1965), depending on the respective situation. Sommer (1969) described it as follows:

> Personal space refers to an area with an invisible boundary surrounding the person's body into which intruders may not come. Like the porcupines in Schopenhauer's fable, people like to be close enough to obtain warmth and comradeship but far enough away to avoid pricking one

another. Personal space is not necessarily spherical in shape nor does it extend equally in all directions... (p.26).

Another definition is proposed by Goffman (1971) who stated that personal space is the 'space surrounding an individual anywhere within which an entering other causes the individual to feel encroached upon, leading him to show displeasure and sometimes to withdraw' (p.29-30).

The issue of personal space is strongly interrelated with the concept of territory. There are, however, important differences between the two (Sommer, 1959). Personal space is portable in contrast to the relatively immobile territory. Boundaries of territories are usually marked and hence visible, boundaries of personal space are always invisible. The human body represents more or less the centre of the personal space, depending on its shape, but not the centre of a territory.

Theoretical approaches to personal space
There exist several theories of personal space. The most dominant approach was proposed by Hall (1966), an anthropologist. He pointed out the use of spatial zones as a means of non-verbal communication (see also 'The Silent Language', 1959) and coined the term 'proxemics', representing the study of man's use of space as a vehicle of communication. He stated that interpersonal distance provides participants and outsiders with information about the nature of the participants' relationship. On the basis of his investigations, Hall described four spatial zones, each divided into a near and a far phase, that indicate different relationships between individuals.

Intimate distance (0-18 inches; 0-45 cm). This distance allows activities with possible body-contact. Individuals interacting in this distance are usually on very close terms. Such interaction with other persons is seen as inappropriate and creates tension and stress.

Personal distance (1.5-4 feet; 45-120 cm). This distance ranges from a near phase within which close people are permitted to a far phase for friends or acquaintances. One has to disagree with Altman and Chemers' (1980) assumption that personal distance can be equated with personal space. Personal distance appears to be a concept more closely defined, whereas personal space represents certainly a wider range of distances, although overlapping to various degrees. Interesting is that people maintain a greater distance from individuals with abnormalities, be it a physical or mental handicap or another social stigma of deviation (Altman, 1975).

Social distance (4-12 feet; 1,2-3,5 m). This distance allows interaction with strangers or the conduct business, when one wants to be in contact with others but not in a close way.

Public distance (12-25 feet and more; 3,5-7m and more). This distance is rarely used for communication between two individuals rather than by a speaker and his audience. The far phase is maintained when meeting a high-status figure.

Hall's data were obtained through interviews and observations of non-contact, middle-class, healthy adults of the Northeast of the United States. Today, almost 30 years later, one can assume that, as times and norms change, American subjects might show slightly different findings. Various studies, however, confirmed that Hall's model applies also to other cultures, although the distances may vary within a predictable range (Altman, 1975).

Influences on personal space
Altman (1975) compiled a vast variety of studies and determined three broad categories of factors that affect personal space:
1 Individual factors like age, race (Winogrond, 1981), upbringing, gender, personality characteristics are named. For example, in Cavallin and Houston's study (1980) aggressive male individuals preferred a greater distance in face-to-face encounters than the normal population. An important factor is the cultural background of an individual. Hall (1966) pointed out the use of space in different cultural contexts (American, English, German, French, Japanese and Arab) and divided them into 'contact' and 'non-contact' cultures. He described, for example, the Germans as more territorial than Americans and as people who take the demarcation of doors seriously. Although this global framework is defended by some research, there are also a number of cross-cultural studies that do not allow such a simplistic generalization. The techniques used in most of those studies, however, cannot be considered objective (Evans and Howard, 1973).
2 Interpersonal factors are represented by the social relationship between individuals. On the basis of research that confirmed the dependence of interaction distances on the degree of acquaintance (for example Little, 1965), Sundstrom and Altman (1976) developed their 'Model of Personal Space and Interpersonal Relationships'. It is organized around three interpersonal situations: (a) ongoing interaction between friends or relatives, (b) interaction between strangers and (c) situations where two strangers do not expect to interact, and the various degrees of comfortable or uncomfortable distances in these situations.
3 Situational factors refer to the impact of settings on the regulation of boundaries.

Intrusion into personal space
There is a considerable body of research based knowledge on individuals' reactions to spatial invasions of others although very little research can be found on the personal experience of the victims. Sundstrom and Altman (1976)

understand spatial invasions as occurring 'when an individual violates norms of interpersonal distance by approaching too closely and the subject does not expect or desire to interact with the potential invader' (p.55). The victim shows signs of discomfort, embarrassment, restlessness and reacts typically with turning, moving away, looking away or flight. From a psychological point of view, too close a distance deprives a person of feelings of autonomy and self-determination (Ingham, 1978). Intrusions can only be tolerated when they occur through high density such as in lifts or overcrowded buses and are involuntarily. Deliberate spatial invasion, however, is seen as seriously aggressive behaviour.

Research on invasion of personal space covers such a wide range as behavioural reaction (Felipe and Sommer, 1966), galvanic skin responses (McBride, King and James, 1965), blood pressure (Hackworth, 1976), stress (Long, 1984), test anxiety (McElroy and Middlemist, 1983) or anger (O'Neal, Brunault, Marquis and Carifio, 1979).

Research methods for studying personal space
The literature shows three general approaches to investigation of personal space: simulation, laboratory and naturalistic methods.

Simulation techniques. Real life is simulated on a model scale. Felt figures, symbols, line drawings or dolls represent people and are put into context according to the subject's perception of interpersonal spacing. One simulation method is the Comfortable Interpersonal Distance Scale (CID) developed by Duke and Novicki (1972). Subjects imagine themselves as the centre of a diagram that shows eight radii emanating from this common point and mark the distance where they think they would feel uncomfortable with the stimulus approaching on a radius. Simulation techniques are easy to administer and can be controlled. Their validity is, however, questionable. They rely on the memory of the subject, his ability to transform actual distances to scaled down distances, and the unconscious aspect of spatial behaviour is not covered.

Laboratory techniques. The so-called 'stop-distance method' is well known, where the distancing process happens in an artificial setting. These methods are also easy to conduct and they overcame the model scale problems of simulation methods. There is, however, still the subject's awareness of the distancing process which might create different behaviour from that seen in real life.

Field/naturalistic techniques. Here personal space is studied in real settings such as libraries or classrooms by unobtrusively observing naturally occurring interpersonal positioning. Sommer's study in 1959 seems to be the first investigation of that kind. Besides the ethical question, there are many uncontrolled variables to deal with and any attempt of measurement raises problems.

15

All these methods, however, are designed to observe behaviour of subjects but not to understand their perceptions and experiences of their body boundaries. Personal space is an important behavioural mechanism in the regulation of social interaction. As the population density grows, the available space becomes less and intrusions into body boundaries become inevitable. This leads us immediately to another aspect interrelated with territory, namely crowding.

Crowding

Crowding is closely linked with the aspects of territoriality and personal space. It has to be seen as a psychological concept and has to be separated from the strictly physical meaning of density, which is simply a measure of people per space unit (Stokols, 1972; cited in Altman, 1975). Crowding, on the other side, can be understood as a personal, subjective reaction and an interpersonal process. Altman (1975) stated that

> …crowding occurs when privacy mechanisms fail to function success-
> fully, causing a person or group to have more interaction with others
> than is desired; that is, achieved privacy is less than desired privacy
> (p.146).

When more social contact occurs than was wanted, one can assume that the boundary control mechanisms (see Altman's model of privacy regulation) failed. The personal space of the individual is invaded leading to physical or psychological stress. The perception of crowding depends like all the other above discussed concepts on personal, social and situational factors.

Research on crowding
There exists a large body of knowledge on crowding obtained by correlational-sociological and by experimental-psychological studies confirming a relationship between crowding and various social or personal problems. Examples can be obtained in reviews by Altman (1975) and Gifford (1987). Potential health problems such as effects on cardiac functions, sweating, and stress were reported in laboratory and field studies. 'If high density has any positive physiological effects … they have not yet been demonstrated' (Gifford, 1987:192).

Coping with crowding
Culturally based aspects of coping with the presence of fellow individuals have already been mentioned before. In studies on response to crowding patterns, aggression or withdrawal were observed. The latter was mainly maintained by looking away, reducing talking or signalling unwillingness to socialize. It is, however, not possible to generalize from these statements that crowding

16

produces aggression or withdrawal. A number of factors determine which coping behaviour will be employed (Altman, 1975).

Embarrassment

Embarrassment is a highly uncomfortable negative experience (Edelmann, 1981) that can vary from minor annoyance to paralysing shock (Apsler, 1975). It is often used synonymously with shame. Buss (1980) and Edelmann (1981), however, distinguished between both concepts and emphasized that shame is an enduring personal feeling carrying a moral burden, whereas embarrassment is a rather momentary experience triggered by an undesired presentation of oneself. It is the public image one is concerned with. Behaviour that is inconsistent with social rules is likely to produce embarrassment (Edelmann, 1985). This public self-awareness has to be learned by children. It is, therefore, hardly surprising that Buss, Iscoe and Buss (1979) demonstrated that children show embarrassment from the age of five. However, because of the research method used – the data were obtained by untrained observers, i.e. parents – the findings have to be treated cautiously, but they nevertheless support the view that embarrassment occurs only when the social self is discredited (Goffman, 1959). It always involves others' awareness of the event. Edelmann (1981) defined three common aspects of embarrassing situations: transgression of a social rule, resultant failure of self-presentation, and loss of self-esteem in the presence of others. Buss (1980) named a number of immediate causes for embarrassment. The one relevant to this study is the breach of privacy with the exposure of the body or parts of it, and with the touch and physical closeness of a person entering the intimate zone (Hall, 1966), situations that occur perpetually in the hospital setting. Lange (1970) discussed this issue under the concept of shame and stressed the experience of a patient who enters the hospital and finds privacy not assured. What people tolerate in hospital seems to differ greatly from what they tolerate in public. It is the nurse's task to observe behaviour displayed by embarrassed individuals. There are several studies on reactions to embarrassment (for example Apsler, 1975). More examples can be obtained from Edelmann (1985). Edelmann and Hampson (1979) determined three types of behaviour: reduction of eye contact, increase of body motion, and speech disturbance, all familiar through the earlier discussion in the section on personal space. Whatever one calls the reaction on breach of privacy and exposure of the self – embarrassment or shame – it seems to be a highly stressful experience for the individual which should be avoided whenever possible.

17

Privacy in hospitals

The ability to maintain the desired level of privacy is a necessary aspect of human life. This section of the literature review will discuss the concepts of privacy, territoriality and personal space applied to the hospital setting. Hospitals are physical surroundings for different groups of people, some are in hospital for a longer period of time as recipients of the services, others are able to leave after finishing an eight-hour shift. All of them are exposed to this setting which is so different from home. Kerr (1985), for example, examined space use, privacy and territoriality among hospital nurses. With respect to the research topic, the patient's privacy will be stressed here alone with a brief review of the perspective of visitors because of their close relationships to the patients visited and because of their role as potential patients. First, the available literature on the topic is examined concerning the major different groups of patients/residents.

Patients/residents in long-term settings – psychiatric institutions

One of the most popular settings for review in the literature on privacy is the psychiatric institution. Brought to mind by Goffman (1961), the degree of self-determination and privacy of residents is described by many authors and examined in many studies.

Privacy in the inmate's world. In his famous book 'Asylums' Goffman (1961) reported his observations in a mental hospital. The inmates suffered an almost complete loss of privacy and of autonomy. Personal possessions were taken away, inspections and physical examinations were carried out at staff's will, sanitary facilities were without doors, and as there were no private territories into which to retreat, observation was continuous. Rosenhan (1973) with seven other pseudopatients confirmed these incidents.

Territoriality and personal space in psychiatric settings. It has long been known that schizophrenic patients prefer larger interpersonal distances (Sommer, 1959). Smith and Cantrell (1988) examined the anxiety occurring due to different distances in the nurse-patient encounter. Interestingly, they found that physical distance was anxiety-provoking only if combined with personal questions, whereas verbal intrusion created anxiety irrespective of the physical distance. Links between interpersonal spacing and nonverbal communication were investigated by McGuire and Polsky (1983) who suggested that individuals may increase or reduce the probability of interactions by altering the inter-individual distance.

Besides personal space, the territorial behaviour of psychiatric patients is another widely discussed topic. Esser, Chamberlain, Chapple and Kline (1965) studied the relationship between a patient's dominance in hierarchy and his

18

territorial behaviour and stated that 'a person's instability in the dominance hierarchy and his possession of a territory are both related to aggressive behaviour' (p.43) and they demonstrated that only 50per cent of the patients used the space available to them. Boettcher (1985) named the social ecological process promoting or restricting access to environmental resources that serve as human need satisfiers, 'boundary marking'. She studied territorial behaviour in the institutionalized elderly and defined three conceptual categories that restrict the patient's privacy and self-determination:

1   delineating space: the mobility of patients is highly controlled by locked units, locked sleeping areas and the unlocked space is permanently under staff control;
2   institutionalizing time: the staff establishes timetables and schedules for sleeping, bathing, eating, locking doors;
3   controlling supplies: clothes, money, food is handed out by staff.

Personal autonomy as a function of privacy (Westin, 1967) can certainly not be maintained under these circumstances. Reporting similar events, particularly the defence of the 'own' chair, Cooper (1984) suggested that based on the knowledge of territoriality 'an attempt should be made, whenever possible, to allow for individual control and enjoyment of personal possessions and private living space, no matter how small or seemingly insignificant' (p.11).

Patient surveys. Major surveys in psychiatric hospitals (Raphael and Peers, 1972; Raphael, 1974) also tried to examine the patient's point of view about the level of privacy. There seems not to be much improvement since Goffman's reports. Even now the lack of a place of one's own, exposure in bathrooms, washrooms, lavatories without doors or locks and washbasins without curtains are much complained about, although the sanitary annexes were less criticized than in comparable studies in general hospitals (Raphael and Peers, 1972). One wonders if this is due to adaptation and resignation through years of stay in such a setting. It is also sometimes not very clear whether authors and respondents mean the same phenomenon when they talk about privacy. The need for one's own territory is expressed through the demand for more single rooms, although companionship and therapeutic interaction in larger wards may be valuable (Shields, Morrison and Hart, 1988).

Lack of privacy is used in institutions to encourage conformity and control behaviour (Schultz, 1977). Morgan (1986) described in her essay about ensuring dignity and self-esteem how vulnerable people become 'once they changed from day clothes into pyjamas' (p.12) and suggested that staff should question if they would accept this situation for themselves, their families or friends. 'Ironically, many psychiatric hospital environments inhibit the very social behaviours that are expressed goals of the hospital's therapeutic programs' (Holahan and Wandersman, 1987:837).

Patients/residents in long-term settings – Nursing homes for elderly

Nursing homes as a second major long-term environment also provide opportunity to examine the residents' privacy. Several authors described ward experiences and recommended practical improvements (Trierweiler, 1978; Tate, 1980; Elliott, 1982; Davis, 1984; Vousden, 1987).

Research based literature covers a wide range of studies, for example about elderly people's perception of body boundary, personal space and body size (Phillips, 1979) or about the fact that territorial marking prevents behavioural deterioration due to lack of privacy (Nelson and Paluck, 1980). Roosa (1982) questioned residents about their understanding of privacy. Solitude was the most chosen definition of privacy with self-evaluation as its most appreciated function. Age was seen in a study of 55 – 88 year old women as by far the most important predictor of preferred personal space (Gioiella, 1978) which contradicted other findings (Johnson, 1979; Geden and Begeman, 1981) that age made no significant difference at all. Gioiella, however, acknowledged that the theory and methodology of her study might have been not appropriate. By confirming feelings of anxiety in 60 – 95 year old residents when their territories were intruded upon, Johnson (1979) supported Allekian's (1973) results. She also stressed, like Allekian, that the lowest anxiety occurred during intrusions caused by nurses when they sat on beds or entered the room without knocking, higher levels of anxiety were reported when residents were intruders. To find out more about personal space in elderly people, Louis (1981) tried to assess personal space boundaries by letting the subjects be approached by other individuals from different angles. It was interesting in this context that their personal space needs were greater laterally than anteriorly, which contradicts common theories that a person is more sensitive to a face-to-face intrusion. Unfortunately, no reasons for these findings were suggested.

Surveys on a larger scale were conducted by Raphael (1979; in 6 hospitals) and Willcocks, Peace and Kellaher (1987; in 100 homes). Violation of residents' sense of privacy occurred mainly in connection with hygiene and elimination but also when too many roommates had to share sleeping quarters or the architectural design made it impossible to spend time alone. That these conditions are far from superseded is shown in a survey of 114 registered homes in the Greater London area (Counsel and Care, 1991). The patient's sense of dignity and privacy is still violated. It seems, for example, still to be common practice that residents have to use a commode in front of their roommates.

The similarities between the respect for privacy in psychiatric institutions and in homes for elderly are worrying. It seems as if people who are not of any apparent use to society are automatically deprived of the basic human right to dignity, respect, autonomy and self-determination.

Privacy in acute care settings

Whereas there was a wide range of literature on privacy in psychiatric institutions or in homes for the elderly, much less can be found on privacy in acute care settings.

Several anecdotal articles acknowledge the problem generally (Davidson, 1990) in a paediatric context (Milligan, 1987), in emergency departments (Johnston, 1988), in the search for patient identification in emergencies (George and Quattrone, 1985), in recovery rooms (Minckley, 1968) or in connection with critically ill patients (Roberts, 1986). Hodgson (1975) examined the topic from a different point of view and stated that it was not financial restraints but prejudice which prevents the establishment of provisions for more privacy. Clade (1989) and Globig (1991) suggested privacy issues merely between the lines.

There seem to be no recent large scale surveys concerning this topic. In Cartwright's (1964) study only 13 per cent of the patients claimed they did not have enough privacy. Ten years later, Raphael (1973) questioned 1348 patients in 10 general hospitals. Besides remarks about the curtains having gaps, the beds being too close, unpleasant smells and sounds being annoying and discussions during examinations being restricted as they were within earshot of others, 100 per cent complained about lack of privacy in sanitary facilities. It would be interesting, to find out how patients today, 20 years later, would respond.

Few studies about privacy in acute care settings were found, all of them conducted in the United States. The first is Allekian's (1973) study of intrusions into territory and personal space as anxiety-producing factors for patients. She interviewed 76 adults in four acute care hospitals with a two-fold questionnaire covering (1) territory and (2) personal space. Some of her results were, for example, that a nurse's entry into the room without knocking was responded to with indifference, whereas someone looking through one's belongings, or removal of one's bed-side table, or opening/closing of one's windows or shades, all without permission, provoked strong reactions. Personal space intrusions did not seem to be as anxiety-producing as one might have assumed. Intrusions into one's territory, however, created strong annoyance. Geden and Begeman (1981) compared personal space preferences (PSP) of 60 hospitalized adults in hospital and in home settings and examined whether these patients assigned different PSP to a family member, a nurse, a doctor, or a stranger. They used a figure-placement technique and an open-ended questionnaire. The results of the study showed that age and sex did not affect the PSP. The PSP was significantly smaller in hospital than in the home. The most interesting findings were that the doctor was placed as close as family members, whereas the nurse was located significantly farther away, the stranger furthest. No difference between nurse and doctor was discerned, when Stratton (1981) replicated this study with 6-18 year old patients. However, considering the disadvantages of simulation-tech-

21

niques, the findings should be viewed cautiously. Schuster (1976a) investigated the meaning of privacy for patients and developed a 'model of interpersonal distancing within hospitalization' based on the needs withdrawal/retreat and disclosure/communication. It is, however, difficult to follow Schuster's arguments because of some inconsistencies in the report, mainly through non-existent definitions and a lack of explanation of the data analysis, aspects also criticized by Brink (1976).

Ward routine as intrusion into patient's privacy
In the reviewed literature many aspects of the daily ward routine are mentioned as intrusive. Only literature on acute care settings was selected for this section. Firstly, invasions of the patient's territory and personal space shall be defined. At the top of the list rank complaints about the inappropriate use of curtains/screens (Cartwright, 1964; Bloch, 1970; Gainsborough, 1970; Raphael, 1973; Oland, 1978; Barron, 1990; Davidson, 1990). This represents, of course, a British point of view as curtains around beds are unknown in most countries. Another important aspect is entering the patient's room without knocking (Bloch, 1970; Allekian, 1973; Oland, 1978; Hayter, 1981; Barron, 1990); entering curtains without warning; and leaving doors open (Barron, 1990; Bloch, 1970) – all issues illustrating the free access to a patient beyond his control. Oland (1978) stressed that the 'professional right of entry does not preclude the need to request a client's permission to invade' (p.122). As an area can only be defined as territory when it has a clear definition (Sebba and Churchman, 1983) – here the patient's room or the space within the curtains – the emotional stress on the holder of the territory that is constantly invaded can easily be understood. Besides the invasion, unauthorized changes within this territory like re/moving furniture, closing or opening windows or shades (Allekian, 1973); borrowing a wheel chair for another patient (Levine, 1968); rearranging objects on the bedside table, and throwing away seemingly worthless articles (Hayter, 1981; Oland, 1978), or rummaging through the patient's personal belongings (Allekian, 1973) are reported as irritating. Also the number of people intruding during a hospital day must be seen as stressful (Gainsborough, 1970; Milligan, 1987). Not only persons who act within a patient's territory are seen as disturbing but also bulky equipment being used for another patient or the fact that beds are too close (Raphael, 1973; Roberts, 1986). Lack of sufficient and lockable space for the safe keeping of personal belongings was reported by Hayter (1981), Meisenhelder (1982), and Roberts (1986). 'Human beings vest something of themselves in personal belongings' as Bryant (1978:63) stated, and he assumed that denying a rightful place for those possessions is damaging. How many nurses have not had the experience of finding private articles such as photos, money, or dentures carefully wrapped and hidden under pillows or bed sheets? Considering the patient's personal space, too close a contact with the nurse (be it through sitting on the bed,

22

touch, or through performing care to intimate areas (Allekian, 1973; Mallon-Palmer, 1980)) must not be assumed to be welcome to every patient. In the most widely used German nursing textbook (Juchli, 1991) only a few lines are dedicated to territoriality.

Besides spatial invasions, violation of a patient's dignity is another topic related to the patient's privacy. It is worth mentioning that the vast majority of articles considered the issues of hygiene and elimination. Exposure of the patient's body during washing and bathing was reported very often and so also were degrading toilet procedure facilities, either on the ward or in the room (e.g. Cartwright, 1964; Gainsborough, 1970; Raphael, 1973; Barron, 1990). Little privacy exists when patients have to give information in front of others or when conversations with doctors or visitors can be overheard through the curtain. Probing and penetrating questions are highly stressful for a patient (Bloch, 1970) forced to produce information. Aasterud (1962) suggested that there are also subtle invasions of privacy of feelings like 'the highly personal questions often asked for no other reason than that of curiosity, and the witnessing of emotions and family situations not normally open to the view of strangers' (p.54). Another threat to patient privacy is – and this might apply especially to individuals who are used to a solitary life – that too many strangers are in a room and that there is no choice of whom one has to sleep next to (Hodgson, 1971; Cantrell, 1978).

Teaching students as a danger to patient's privacy
Another situation in which patient privacy is threatened occurs when students of the health care professions have to be taught using the patient as an audio-visual aid. Almost nothing can be found about this topic in the literature on clinical teaching. Hinchliff (1989) merely mentioned the patient's need for privacy and suggested the use of a separate venue if confidential information in relation to nursing care is to be transmitted. One can imagine the difficult situation a patient experiences who has to relate the history in front of a group of students or who undergoes examinations (e.g. in gynaecology), watched by a number of curious spectators. It is, however, not only the obvious exposure to strangers that causes concern. Even if a patient is spared embarrassment and, for example, is interviewed or filmed in a small studio, these audio-visual aids can be duplicated and distributed beyond the patient's control (Cantrell, 1978).

Touch as nursing action
There exists a now sizeable literature dealing with touch as a nursing measure. Fromm-Reichmann (cited in De Augustinis, Isami and Kumler, 1963) stated that the need for physical contact is innate and that physical and emotional disturbances are caused by lack of physical contact. She acknowledged cultural differences and pointed out that

...among the people in the middle and upper social strata in our Western culture, physical loneliness has become a specific problem, since the culture is governed by so many obsessional taboos with regard to people's touching one another or having their physical privacy threatened in other ways (p.275).

Culture largely dictates the employment of touch (Hall and Whyte, 1976). The change in the use of touch from archaic man to modern Western culture is illustrated by Burton and Heller (1964). Although in Western culture touch is permitted only to close people, nurses seem to be socially exempted from this rule by their professional function, to act as a mother surrogate and therefore touch another person who is often a total stranger (Mercer, 1966).

Touch is a very important aspect of nursing care and contributes to the patient's welfare (Loscin, 1984). It is employed as 'therapeutic touch' to support or even substitute traditional treatment (Heidt, 1981; 1991).

There are several studies on touch in the nurse-patient relationship, for example, about the application of touch during labour and delivery (Lorensen, 1983), the decrease of anxiety levels through the use of therapeutic touch (Heidt, 1991), patients' perceptions of touch used by nurses (Mulaik, Megenity, Cannon, Chance, Cannella, Garland and Gilead, 1991). Oliver and Redfern (1991) developed an observation schedule to record and classify touch in the nurse-patient encounter.

Touch is the first and most fundamental means of communication (De Augustinis et al., 1963; Durr, 1971; Barnett, 1972; Weiss, 1979). Because of its physical intimacy, it is the most powerful communication channel and the most carefully guarded and regulated (Thayer, 1988). Barnett (1972) reviewed the literature on the topic, also in relation to nursing, and defined several concepts of touch: mechanics of communication, touch as a means of communicating, touch as a basis for establishing communication, touch as a means of communicating emotions, and touch as a means of communicating ideas. There is – at least in the nurse-patient relationship – a danger of misinterpretation (Mercer, 1966; Levine, 1968; Loscin, 1984; Oliver and Redfern, 1991). This risk of misinterpreting touch by either the patient or the nurse was found to be 50 per cent (De Augustinis et al., 1963). As both touch and spatial behaviour are seen as non-verbal communication, it is curious that De Augustinis et al. – although as early as 1963 – did not mention the obvious link between the two concepts. Neither do more recent authors (Heidt, 1981, 1991; Lorensen, 1983). Others, like Durr (1971), Barnett (1972), Loscin (1984) and Oliver and Redfern (1991) include it at least in some way.

Two investigations, however, cover the impact of touch on the patient's personal space. Lane's descriptive study (1989) was an attempt to determine if male and female adult surgical clients' and female registered nurses' perception about intrusions of patients' territory and personal space in the hospital differed. She employed a questionnaire derived from Allekian's (1973) Likert scale, used to measure patients' responses to intrusions. Male patients showed more positive emotions than female patients, contrary to the nurses' expectations. Allekian's study also showed that for female patients touch was not welcome. Another study focused on the relationship of touch to aggressive behaviour in a nursing home (Marx, Werner and Cohen-Mansfield, 1989). They found that touch decreased physically nonaggressive behaviour, like repetitious mannerisms, but increased aggressive behaviours, and they suggested that residents may interpret touch as a violation of their personal space.

It seems that the concept of territoriality and personal space has to be given more consideration when the use of touch in a therapeutic setting is recommended, especially as research based knowledge is rather scarce.

Privacy dependent on social class
Bryant (1978) assumed that in private hospitals there would be a greater concern for patients' privacy than in public hospitals. It seems that 'the amount of space a person has rights to often is related to his personal significance or financial status' (Pluckhan, 1968:393). This view is shared by Tungpalan (1982). Bloch (1970) hypothesized that 'within the health profession, there may be a tendency to invade the privacy of people of those classes below us, with a hesitation to invade the privacy of those in higher classes' (p.264) and she recommended more research into this aspect. For Roberts (1986) the advantage of social importance goes even beyond space:

> The more socially prominent the patient, the more access he has to physical territory, in terms of both quality and quantity. In addition, his personal territory may extend throughout the hospital via connections with the significant people within hospital hierarchy (p.121).

Privacy has to be paid for dearly but it is more the private room than special treatment that is desired (Davidson, 1990). A patient, however, can expect that more advantages come with the private room – for example, more suitable waking times (Bauer, 1991) or better food. One reason why some people want private treatment that is expensive because less 'public' might be the fear of losing oneself as a private individual in the system (Cantrell, 1978). It would be interesting to find out why doctors or senior nurses almost always choose single rooms for themselves. Privacy in patient care should not be improved by simply driving the patient to buy a bed, but by planning future wards with privacy in mind, an improvement independent of the individual's financial possibilities, as Gainsborough (1970) recommended.

Patients expect less privacy in hospitals
Patient autonomy is often suggested as essential in nursing care, and 'patient-centred' care is a popular notion. However, nursing will always be intrusive due to

25

its very nature. Personal boundaries will always be invaded to some degree (Schuster, 1976a). Sommer and Dewar (1963) stated that 'nurses and physicians appear to have no reluctance about intruding into [a patient's] personal space. They tend to view his body as an object lacking any kind of aura or sanctity' (p.323). Tungpalan (1982) saw the nurses' uniform as a kind of passport to invade a patient's personal territory. Indeed, in some professional relationships invasions of privacy are accepted due to the role of the invader (Ingham, 1978). Based on their findings, Allekian (1973) and Johnson (1979) suggested that a person entering a hospital anticipates a certain amount of staff intrusion and is psychologically prepared, as he must feel he has not much control over the staff's actions. This anticipation is illustrated by a patient's answer to the question about privacy in his hospital: 'You go into hospital to get better. You don't go in to have a good time or to have privacy' (Cartwright, 1964:60). Durr (1971) provided similar examples of patients who believe that the intimate zone is an appropriate area for nurses to occupy. There are assumptions that patients cope by treating witnesses of intrusions as 'non-persons' (Emerson, 1973; Rosenhan, 1973; Schultz, 1977).

Privacy as a cultural aspect of nursing
Hall (1966) pointed out the varied personal space needs in different cultures, and Altman (1975) incorporated cultural practices in his dialectic model of privacy regulation. Literature examined in this chapter represents almost exclusively American or British culture. Although there are common aspects between the two cultures, the different preferences on size of patient's rooms – for example, single rooms in the USA, large rooms in Britain – is astonishing. The significance of culture became a more and more important issue in nursing and led to terms like 'ethnonursing' (Leininger, 1985) or 'transcultural nursing'. Extensive literature can be obtained, for example, in Dobson (1991). However, privacy is rarely mentioned in this connection. Roosa (1982) assumed cautiously that the meaning of privacy and privacy-seeking behaviour may vary with cultural backgrounds. Only Giger and Davidhizar (1990) emphasized the aspect of comfort in the nurse's responsiveness to the patient's spatial needs and stated 'to give culturally appropriate care, an understanding of interpersonal space is important for the nurse' (p.11). Barron (1990) provided an interesting comparison of nurses' attitudes to offering privacy and of patients' responses in Sweden and in Britain. It seemed as if British nurses concentrate their efforts in providing privacy almost exclusively on the curtains around the bed. Despite the fact that Germans seem to have strong territorial and personal space needs (Hall, 1966; Evans and Howard, 1973) a search in international indices produced not a single German text about patient privacy.

'Unpopular' Patients
A hospital admission is a major event in a person's life. He has to leave a familiar home and people and stay for a period of time in a new and usually strange

26

environment with strange people, procedures, regulations and so on. Hospital routine is arranged for the convenience of nurses and doctors to enable the smooth running of the work, not for the benefit of the patients (Freidson, 1970). A unilateral adaptation is expected of the clients (Boettcher, 1985)and is remarkably met by the patients' ability to adapt to hospital life when they are ill and when it is really necessary (Cantrell, 1978). There are, however, a number of patients who do not perform according to the norms for various reasons. Several authors (Sarosi, 1968; Lorber, 1979; Stockwell, 1984) dealt with this aspect of 'good' and 'bad' patients. In Stockwell's study, for example, 74 per cent of written and 65 per cent of oral comments were collected that labelled patients as unpopular because they were demanding, complaining, bad-tempered or uncooperative.

Bearing in mind the emotional disturbance that can occur when an individual's personal space is invaded, one cannot help wondering if these patients were in fact not bad patients but harassed patients, or, as Mallon-Palmer (1980) assumed:

> ...he may not be 'demanding', 'uncooperative', 'eccentric' or 'maladjusted', he may just be silently resentful about invasions of his private personal space (p.37).

Helber (1991) did not mention intrusion of personal space as a cause of the 'difficult' patient's behaviour. Violated privacy played only a small role in a study on 'difficult' elderly patients (English and Morse, 1988). MacGregor (1967) recognized the cultural variable in the interpretation of 'uncooperative' behaviour but she did not refer to the issues of this current study. Viguers acknowledged in 1959, when investigations into personal space had just started, that the change of environment, examinations, questions and procedures would violate a patient's sense of privacy and cause emotional disturbance. Analyses from this perspective (Schuster, 1976a,b; Louis, 1981) support the link between the intrusion into the patient's personal space and his response. The behaviour in question is, for example, closing the eyes, posting barriers, turning to the wall, pretending to sleep, looking or moving away, not answering questions, refusing procedures or complaining (Hayter, 1981; Roberts, 1986). Patients who – on the other hand – see the hospital environment as nurses' territory display 'good' behaviour (Tungpalan, 1982). However, an extensive literature review by Kelly and May (1982) did not mention at all the connection between intrusions into privacy and the unappreciated behaviour of patients.

The staff's reaction to such deviant behaviour is interesting. Lorber (1979) found that in 69 per cent of the cases drugs were used to handle the situation. Robinson (1979) stated that 'clinical staff often do not observe the patient's need for privacy until the latter has escalated provocative and sometimes maladaptive behaviours to achieve it' (p.20). Gioiella (1978) took the same point of view in her study of personal space of the elderly when she suggested that 'health care professions have misinterpreted a preference for more personal space in the elderly as withdrawal or disengagement' (p.43). Non-verbal behaviour as privacy regulation (Altman, 1975) seems not to be recognized. One must question if there is any knowledge or awareness existing about patients' territorial behaviour.

Ward environment

It has long been known that there is a relationship between an individual's environment and his degree of well-being. The therapeutic benefit of physical surroundings was illustrated by Canter and Canter (1979). The question remains if the current ward environment is indeed beneficial for the patient's well-being; whether, for instance, the ward design is suitable to protect a patient's sense of privacy. Cultural differences explain, for example, the preferences of patients in the USA for more single or double bedrooms whereas British patients seem to prefer the company in larger rooms (Royal Commission on the National Health Service, 1979). German patients seem also to like one to three bedded rooms better (Clade, 1989). The hospital setting must serve many users and functions. When it was stated above that the hospital regulations are made for the staff's convenience to facilitate a well organized work performance, the same can be said about the design of wards. Seelye (1982) represented this point of view when he assumed that factors which enable the best possible care may become more important than questions of privacy.

A number of studies cover the ward environment and its impact on health care workers. One of the first of this kind was conducted by the Nuffield Provincial Hospital Trusts (1955). Its findings were important in creating suitable designs for hospital purposes. Over the years many research based suggestions were made. Jaco (1979) examined patient care in radial and angular units on the assumption that the shape and arrangement of the ward has an impact on the behaviour of staff and patients. Nurses liked the circular wards more because they facilitated easier surveillance and meant less walking, the patients, however, had less privacy as a result of this design. In a recent study in Holland (Meijer, 1992) privacy was seen as one factor influenced by the ward environment. Citations of additional studies could be extended at length but more examples can be obtained in extensive literature reviews by Kenny and Canter (1979), Reizenstein (1982), Seelye (1982) and Williams (1988). Most of the literature on ward environment has one point in common: it scrutinizes the topic from an outsider's point of view and thereby concentrates mainly on work organization related to nurses, doctors and other health care workers (for example, Rosengren and DeVault, 1963; Neufert, 1979; Canter, 1984). Very little can be found considering the patient in the hospital setting, nothing about qualitative data covering the patient's perceptions of his physical surroundings.

Perhaps the most extraordinary aspect of the literature of hospital architecture is that relatively few planners and researchers have ever

28

considered the patient's point of view or sought his ideas or opinions (Wainwright, 1985:49).

Shumaker and Reizenstein (1982) were confronted with the same problem when they wrote about environmental factors that affect inpatient stress and saw their work finally as a suggestion for further extensive research. They defined several sources of stress, one of which was the continuous violation of the ability to maintain control over privacy or personal space (also stated by Sommer and Dewar, 1963), a function critical to a person's health and well-being (Altman, 1975). They stated that

> ...due to their need to 'get the job done' and sometimes to a learned insensitivity to patient needs, medical and nursing staff do not always respect a patient's need for visual or acoustical privacy, or for a patient's need to regulate social interaction (pp.206-7).

Kornfeld (1977) assumed that the reason lay in the staff's need to develop psychological defences to enable them to cope with their own problems, an issue discussed earlier by Menzies (1970). In fairness to the staff one can argue that knowledge about territoriality and personal space applied to the hospital setting is very limited and not part of the educational curriculum.

Referring to the lack of consideration of patient's needs by hospital architects, Shumaker and Reizenstein (1982) suggested that patient control of privacy should be a design principle, practised, for example, by Ritter and von Eiff (1988). Modern ward lay-outs (for example Hubeli, 1989) try to meet these needs.

Visitor's privacy
Zimring, Carpman and Michelson (1987) identified three reasons why hospital visitors are only rudimentarily targeted in the literature:
1 Although large in number, visitors are in the hospital for limited periods of time.
2 Their needs conflict with needs of more powerful groups (staff, patients).
3 Only very little information about the needs and preferences of hospital visitors exists.

However, visitors are an important population because of their psychosocial support for patients, their role as links with the 'outside' world, and because they perform tasks in patient care. Applied to the USA, 'visitors are natural targets for hospitals' marketing interests because they themselves are potential patients and because they may influence friends' or family's choice of health-care facilities' (Zimring et al., 1987:938). A visit to a hospital represents for many people an uncomfortable experience because of their worries about the sick patient, the disruption of the daily routine and the unfamiliar environment. Visitors cannot – like patients – claim a certain territory of their own, except when their patient occupies a private room. A large study at the University of Michigan Hospital (cited in Zimring et al., 1987) defined four environmental design issues relevant to hospital visitors: (1) orientation, (2) physical comfort, (3) privacy and personal territory, and (4) symbolic meaning. In the present study the third issue was of greatest concern. In the above mentioned study about half the visitors of patients in semiprivate or multiple bed rooms would have liked more acoustic privacy which was also extended to the telephone, supporting Cartwright (1964). The privacy of a patient is closely linked with the privacy of his visitor/s. Violations seem to have a negative effect on both parties alike.

More research on patient's privacy is required
This chapter outlined some of the main theoretical frameworks of privacy, territoriality, personal space and other privacy-related concepts. Some of these concepts are rather philosophical and theoretical and lack the support of empirical data. Others claim to be research-based. Many of those studies, however, depended on very specific conditions in a laboratory, applied to very specific situations only, and/or utilized the popular but unrealistic study population of young university students. It has yet to be proven that generalizations can be made from those findings.

Summarizing the aspects of the current base of theoretical development, one can assume that privacy is an individual's basic right and basic need. If this individually perceived need, which depends on several factors, is not met, a number of regulation mechanisms are employed. If unsuccessful, serious psychological and physiological disturbances have to be expected.

Using this base as a starting point, the present research aims at clarifying if part of this theory applies to a group of people who, due to their circumstances, are prone to constant violation of their privacy but are limited in their choice of defensive behaviour. Patients go to hospital to get better. This aim is in danger if it is true that the failure of maintaining one's desired degree of privacy has a detrimental effect on mental and physical health. There is no better way of finding out but asking the individuals concerned if they support or refute the current theoretical knowledge.

The extensive anecdotal literature indicates that patients' privacy in hospitals is an acknowledged problem. The urgent need for further research is illustrated as well. Only a few studies have been conducted, from which countless questions arise (Bloch, 1970; Allekian, 1973; Geden and Begeman, 1981; Kerr, 1982; Meisenhelder, 1982; Barron, 1990; Davidson, 1990). Up to now most of these remain unanswered. Most of those detailed questions, however, have to do with displayed behaviour, practical aspects or nurses' attitudes. The patients' own experience of privacy – as a starting point – is considered only by Rawnsley (1980) who acknowledged the need for a descriptive and phenomenological approach to the study of privacy. This stance was taken when the present study was planned. It seemed to be logical to start at the beginning and ask patients how they felt about their privacy in hospital. It was hoped that the findings will form a basis for an inductive theory development which eventually can be tested deductively. The interpretation of the data should give some insight into patients' ways of feeling, and hopefully come up with some structured evidence that might fit the theoretical deliberations offered in the literature. Bearing in mind that no study on patient's privacy could be found within the German context, this present investigation seemed warranted.

2 Method 1 – interviews

The previous chapter explored the literature on patient privacy. This chapter identifies the methodology of the first step of the data collection and gives explanations about the choice of the phenomenological method used at this stage.

Aims of the research

A number of interesting questions arise from the literature discussed in the previous chapter. The focus of the study was patients' privacy in an acute care setting. Its purpose was to evolve a structural description of the experience 'privacy in hospitals' as lived by the patients. The defined research objectives were

1   to examine patients' perception of their privacy in hospital with particular reference to exposure of identity, exposure of body, territoriality and personal space using semi-structured interviews;
2   to establish if trends emerging from the interview can be found in a larger sample by using a Likert-scale questionnaire;
3   to determine a rank order of privacy-invading events.

These three objectives resembled the three stages of the data collection.

Definitions

For the purpose of this study, privacy was defined as 'the freedom to determine when, under which circumstances and to what extent personal information is shared with or withheld from others' – which is a combination of a variety of definitions of privacy. This definition was purposefully broad in order to define a focus rather than limits to the study. Patients were defined as adults who were at least three days in hospital and were able to comprehend the questions and provide an opinion.

The research setting

The study was carried out in a 502-bed acute care hospital with a large rural catchment area in the south east of the Federal Republic of Germany which was at the same time a teaching hospital of a big Southern university. The hospital consisted of an old complex of buildings constructed between 1928 and 1965, and a new wing opened in 1987. Two medical and two surgical wards were used because these are the most typical wards in hospitals. The oncological ward was included as well because it had the attributes of a medical ward.

Design of the study – first stage: interviews

The qualitative research

The goal of qualitative research is not measurement but knowledge and understanding of phenomena (Leininger, 1985). This kind of study is commonly used when the purpose is to gain insight in a field where little is known (Field and Morse, 1985), in this case patients' perceptions of privacy. The qualitative approach explores the meanings which people assign to aspects of the social world. It can be used for phenomena 'which cannot be broken down without losing sight of the whole' (Bockmon and Riemen, 1987). Qualitative findings often illuminate quantitatively gathered data (Goodwin and Goodwin, 1984; Knafl and Howard, 1984; Polit and Hungler, 1989).

Phenomenology

The philosophy and its historical perspective. The phenomenological movement appeared as a reaction to the denigration of philosophical knowledge and the objectification of human beings (Omery, 1983) that was based on the natural scientific approach of positivism. Positivism is a branch of philosophy developed by Auguste Comte (1798-1857) which recognizes only what can be observed by senses. Quantitative conceptualization of physical objects, however, leaves no room for human experience. Wilhelm Wundt founded in 1879 the 'scientific' psychology utilizing experimental methodology. But he also eliminated experience 'in an attempt to legitimize the science of psychology' (Knaak, 1984:108).

The importance of perception and personal experience was valued in the descriptive phenomenology whose forerunner was the German Brentano (1838-1917). His student Husserl (1859-1938) developed it further and is seen as the founder of (transcendental) phenomenology, which meant for him 'the rigorous and unbiased study of things as they appear so that one might come to an essential understanding of human consciousness and experience' (Valle, King and Halling, 1989:6), a thought represented in his appeal '*zu den Sachen selbst*' (to the things themselves) (Husserl, 1976). He was concerned with the everyday experience described in everyday language. Stumpf (1848-1936) was convinced that experience has to be studied by all possible methods and founded experimental phenomenology, a concept that is on first sight incompatible with the philosophy. The second important German philosopher and the one who influenced the second (existential) branch of phenomenology was Heidegger (1889-1976). His work *Sein und Zeit* (Heidegger, 1929) is said to have inspired the later French phenomenologists (Cohen, 1987), like Sartre (1905-1980) who coined the phrase 'phenomenological existentialism' (Sartre, 1943), or Merleau-Ponty (1908-1961) who stressed the importance of the individual's perception (Merleau-Ponty, 1962). The essence of phenomenology is that 'it devotes itself to the study of how things appear to the consciousness or are given in experience' (Giorgi, 1986:6).

The phenomenological method

Based on this philosophy is the phenomenological approach to the study of human experience. Van den Berg (1972a) called the method 'a way of observing, new in science; new, for instance, in psychology, not at all new in general life' (p.77). The purpose of the phenomenological method is to study lived experience from the perspective of the experiencing person. Its goal is to describe the experience of the phenomenon under study, not to generate opinions or theories (Parse, Coyne and Smith, 1985; Field and Morse, 1985; Munhall and Oiler, 1986; Oiler, 1986; Wertz, 1986). The emphasis lies on the description as the main technique (Giorgi, 1975) or, as Spinelli (1989) puts it: 'describe, don't explain' (p.17). Spinelli's 'Equalization Rule' has certainly to be considered which said that initially one should avoid to place described items in a hierarchy but treat them as having equal significance.

The life-world as focus of investigation Life-world is described as 'the world as it is lived by the person and not the hypothetical external entity separate from or independent of him or her' (Valle et al., 1989:9). Van den Berg (1972b), for example, described the life-world of a patient and the patient's entire experiences as they were lived by him and not observed and interpreted by others. The life-world is lived by all of us before any explanations or theoretical interpretations are made (Giorgi, 1975). According to Schutz (1970) it is a biographically determined situation based upon a stock of experiences that function as a scheme of reference. Hagan (1986) emphasized that in order to study a person's lived experience one has to get as close as possible to this individual's understanding of his/her life-world 'rather than amassing facts as they appear to the researcher

34

with her assumed access to objective reality' (p.347). In order to be able to do this a researcher needs to have certain attitudes and skills. He/she has to immerse empathetically into the described world, dwell upon the situation, magnify and amplify seemingly unimportant things, take a step back and examine the description with great interest whereby he/she directs the attention from the described object to the meaning it has for the describing subject. The researcher also has to be able to recognize and use an 'existential baseline', and among other things, reflect on his or her judgement, make distinctions, recognize relations and use appropriate language to express the findings (Wertz, 1983, 1985). A certain amount of experience is also of great importance or at least the opportunity to observe an experienced researcher (Spiegelberg, 1982).

Bracketing. An important process in the phenomenological method is called 'bracketing' or 'epoché' (ἐποχή), a term coined by Husserl (1976), which is derived from the Greek 'to pause and look for the truth' (Ritter, 1972). In order to view the phenomena under study clearly and 'to experience them freshly' (Giorgi, 1986:16), it is necessary to make a serious effort to set aside all prejudices, biases, beliefs, assumptions, and conceptualized experience one has. Schutz (1970) suggested that it is only after bracketing that some very important structures of consciousness can be made accessible. The process of bracketing is dynamic; as one starts bracketing, more preconceptions emerge that need to be bracketed. The world as it is observed is reduced to the world of pure phenomena, this is why the term 'reduction' is often used synonymously for bracketing (Valle et al., 1989). Bracketing is an extremely difficult task. Complete reduction is impossible (Merleau-Ponty, 1962). Spinelli (1989) argued less rigorously when he said 'although it may well be impossible for us to bracket all biases and assumptions, we are certainly capable of bracketing a substantial number of them' (p.17).

Oiler (1986) recommended a review of the relevant literature after the data are collected. This seems, however, rarely possible as a researcher has to be familiar with the available literature before deciding which aspect of the topic he/she is going to investigate. It is obvious that the process of 'sense-making' during a literature review puts the researcher even more in a position to bracket all those interpretations when it comes to data analysis.

Is total bracketing really desirable?. If it was possible to set aside all one's own views, one might wonder what is left of the researcher's self to interpret the data in a sensitive way. Would not the alternative be to provide the reader with the verbatim transcripts and let him make sense of it? An interesting dialogue on bracketing in Morse (1991) discusses this very problem, where many different points of views on this topic are highlighted.

The importance of the phenomenological method for nursing. Due to the nature of nursing, a nurse is very close to a person who is ill and in crisis. This closeness provides unique access to a patient's experience (Munhall and Oiler, 1986) and should, therefore, be used more to gain a better understanding of a patient's life-world. Swanson-Kaufman (1988) justified phenomenological nursing research by stating

> ...since nursing practice involves diagnosing and treating human responses to actual and potential health problems, and since humans respond as whole persons, knowledge of the lived experience of health and healing are legitimate topics of nursing inquiry (p.97).

Parse et al. (1985) shared this view when they called any human circumstance related to health a phenomenon worthy of investigation in nursing science. However, it is important not only to understand a patient's experience (Davis, 1978; Oiler, 1982; Knaak, 1984; Pallikkathayil and Morgan, 1991) but also to utilize this understanding, i.e. its application to practice (Lynch-Sauer, 1985).

As the traditional scientific research approach was found to be too restrictive, more and more nurse researchers are using a phenomenological method (Omery, 1983). One example is Field's (1981) study about the experience of giving an injection, and a more recent investigation was conducted on the lived experience of health in the oldest of the elderly (Wondolowski and Davis, 1991). The present study aims to utilize the phenomenological approach to describe the lived experience of privacy as perceived by hospitalized patients.

Reliability and validity in qualitative research

The results of qualitative research are often seen as lacking reliability and validity. 'If psychoanalytic and humanistic approaches are mentioned in a discussion of reliability, it is usually to point out their unreliability according to accepted scientific standards' (Wertz, 1986:182). Colaizzi (1978) pointed out that 'if only observable, duplicable and measurable definitions have psychological validity, then a crucial dimension of the human psychological existence, namely, experience, is eliminated from the study of human psychology – and this is done in the name of objectivity' (p.51).

Reliability refers to the extent to which a study may be replicated. External reliability is achieved when researchers replicating a study with the same methods obtain the same results. When multiple investigators agree within one study, internal reliability is obtained. Considering the nature of qualitative research, the subjectivity of the researcher/s cannot be eliminated. Hycner (1985) argued that this subjectivity allows for an 'approach that is most comprehensive and faithful to the phenomenon'. It follows that it would be unrealistic to reason that only one interpretation is legitimate while others are mere distortions (Wertz, 1986). Qualitative research has to do with the perception of human beings concerning certain events in certain settings. 'Because unique situations cannot be reconstructed precisely, even the most exact replication of research methods may fail to produce identical results' (LeCompte and Goetz, 1982:35). Thorndike (1963) stated that to maximize the prediction of socially useful events 'it might be advantageous to sacrifice a little precision in order to gain a greater amount of scope' (p.291). He believed that precision and high reliability are means rather than ends.

Validity is generally defined as the degree of accuracy to which an instrument measures what it is intended to measure (LeCompte and Goetz, 1982; Kvale, 1983). Rosenbaum (1988) distinguished instrument validity, internal validity and external validity. Internal validity is the extent to which findings are genuine representations of some reality. It can be argued that Rosenbaum's instrument validity is in fact part of internal validity. Hycner (1985) suggested several validity checks: (1) participants check whether the findings are valid for them; (2) the researcher has to evaluate whether the findings appear to be true; (3) findings have to be evaluated by a research committee; (4) findings have to be checked against the current literature, and (5) findings have to be submitted to the scientific and lay community.

External validity refers to the degree to which generalizations may be drawn from the results. As the sample in qualitative research is usually small and rarely randomly selected from a wider population, qualitative findings cannot be generalized but rather compared and translated to other groups (LeCompte and Goetz, 1982). In the strict sense the results apply only to the interviewed informant, but 'in the process of even investigating the experience of one unique individual we can learn much about the phenomenology of human being in general' (Hycner, 1985:295). The fidelity to the data is important, not how close one has got to experimental control (Hagan, 1986). Therefore, as Burch (1989) wrote, phenomenology has its own 'narrative rigor' (p.211).

The interview as a qualitative method of data collection
Kvale (1983) defined the purpose of an interview as 'description and under-standing of the meaning of themes in the life-world of the interviewee'(p.180). He emphasized a number of aspects: the interview is centred on the inter-viewee's life-world; it seeks to understand the meaning of phenomena; it is qual-itative, descriptive, and specific; it avoids presuppositions; it is focused on certain themes; it is open for ambiguities, and changes; it depends upon the sensitivity of the interviewer; it takes place in an interpersonal interaction, and it may be a positive experience. Rich, detailed, valid and reliable data are provided (Lofland and Lofland, 1984; Marshall and Rossman, 1989). Taylor and Bogdan (1984) interpreted the interview as an 'encounter between researcher and informants' perspectives on their lives, experience or situations as expressed in their own words' (p.77). Its design is, according to Burgess (1984), based on the knowledge the researcher has of a social situation.

Brenner, Brown and Canter (1985) identified some advantages of interviews: (1) misunderstandings on both parts can be checked immediately through negotiations, (2) rapid, immediate response, and (3) extensive data. One of the disadvantages is the opportunity for bias because of the face-to-face contact – for example, the individual tries to please the investigator or holds back private or embarrassing thoughts. However, Pomeroy (1963) assumed that embarrassment was no problem when the following requirements were met: the research was important, needed, and useful to others; the information given was kept in confidence and the interviewer was not judging the subjects. Hutchinson and Wilson (1992) defined possible validity threats in scheduled semi-structured interviews in the questions themselves, in the timing of the interview, in the interviewer's and/or respondent's behaviour, and in the process of recording.

Development of the interview guide
The purpose of this study was to explore and describe patients' perceptions of their privacy during the stay in hospital. No comprehensive tool for investigating the perception of privacy has yet been developed. Interviews seem to be a reasonable method for an initial exploration of a subject's lived experience, especially when no previous knowledge of the topic is available. In order to reach this goal, a semi-structured interview guide was designed. This tool was chosen because it focuses on a certain type of information (Kvale, 1983) but the questions can be modified to fit each respondent (Denzin, 1978). The guide ensures that key topics are discussed with all participants and serves, therefore, as a reminder (Taylor and Bogdan, 1984). Waltz, Strickland and Lenz (1991) provided a procedure for developing interview schedules.

Apart from legal considerations which are not covered in this study, intrusion of privacy seems to exist only when the individual is aware of it (McCloskey, 1971; Ingham, 1978). Therefore, it was decided to include only items a patient can actually perceive during his stay in hospital. Open access to computer data that is unknown to the patient would, for example, not enter the pool of questions. The interview guide covered topics based on likely areas of concern described in the literature and on the researcher's personal experience and was divided into the following categories:
1 General aspects
2 Exposure (visual, acoustical)
3 Territoriality
4 Personal space
Additionally, utilizing Schatzman and Strauss's (1973) advice of 'posing the ideal', the patients were asked what they would change if they could do so, to round up the picture of their response. At the end of the interview guide, a list of ten privacy-invading situations was added for patients to rank the items according to the seriousness of intrusion (see Chapter 6). The interview-guide was discussed with several staff of the hospital to establish content validity.

A fresh copy of the interview guide was used for taking field notes and as a memory device (Lofland and Lofland, 1984). At the top of this sheet, personal data were noted such as age, sex, stay in hospital, mobility, number of beds in room. The sheet was used afterwards as a cover for the transcribed interview.

Sampling
Sampling is the process of selecting a part of the population to represent the entire population (Polit and Hungler, 1987). In quantitative research random sampling allows for a certain degree of generalization. The nature of qualitative research does not allow this degree of generalization. LeCompte and Goetz (1982) stated that for this kind of research comparability and translatability are more important.

Non-probability sampling serves the purpose to select subjects who can function as informants for a particular research approach. 'The point of subject selection is to obtain richly varied descriptions, not to achieve statistical generalization' (Polkinghorne, 1989:48). There are two demands of selection: (1) the subject has experience with the topic under investigation, and (2) the subject is able to describe this experience sufficiently (Colaizzi, 1978; Polkinghorne, 1989).

Convenience sampling was used in choosing patients for the interviews. This method of sampling means that subjects are included in the study because they are readily available (Burns and Grove, 1987). The disadvantage of this method is that one cannot tell how representative it is (Smith, 1981). As the researcher approached the subjects, bias was probably not so significant as it would have been the other way round.

In a former study (Bauer, 1991) effects of group pressure amongst patients could be observed. Witnessing another person volunteer or refuse to volunteer strongly influences potential participants (Rosnow and Rosenthal, 1970). This aspect was, therefore, taken into consideration when the subjects were approached.

To select a sufficient number of participants was not the only problem. Other aspects had to be borne in mind. Due to the voluntary nature of participation, one can question if data gained from people who *are* willing to share their opinions apply to the rest of the population and are, therefore, valid. This study, however, had a different purpose as it emphasizes the importance of the understanding of an individual's meaning of his life-world. Another issue is the possibility that a subject tries to be a 'good' subject and wants to please the interviewer (Dean and Whyte, 1958) by telling her what she probably wants to hear. On the other side, fear of reprisal through staff (Nehring and Geach, 1973) or the anxiety to appear ungrateful through critical comments could influence interviewees' responses.

It was planned to interview 15-20 patients for approximately one hour at a time convenient for the subject. Both sexes were included because of a possible occurrence of specific differences in the findings. This sample size was seen by Wilson and Hutchinson (1991) as sufficient for this purpose. The number of subjects depended on the collected data. When they became repetitious, collecting more data would not have been very productive (Parse et al., 1985).

39

The initial idea was to interview about ten patients on a surgical and about ten on a medical ward. The wards proposed by the hospital management were unfortunately located in a very new building. It was, therefore, decided to extend the study to other medical and surgical wards and an oncological ward in the old part of the hospital. The age of the patients was between 21 and 83 years. Nine women and eleven men participated. Generally, female patients were not that eager to take part in the study.

The decision to approach only patients on their third to fifth day of stay could not be upheld as it was difficult to find enough patients in a relatively short time. It was felt to be more important that patients should be interviewed while still in hospital, and not after discharge, reducing the risk of fallible memory (Salsberry, 1989).

Ethical implications

Ethical aspects in qualitative research were considered, for example, by Ramos (1989), in interviewing, particularly by Smith (1992). A researcher not only has the responsibility to search for knowledge but also to take account of the effects of his work on the subjects (Bulmer, 1982). 'When privacy is investigated, to some extent it is also invaded' (Rawnsley, 1980:30). This was considered while conducting the data collection. It meant practically that the subjects were well-informed about the project, the voluntary nature of the participation and the confidentiality of data. Consent was carefully obtained and the rights of the subjects were protected during the study. Besides behaviour obligatory to general politeness, consideration of subjects' personal space and territoriality was now even more in the researcher's mind. The research topic itself did not imply potential risks for the subjects.

Pilot study

Pilot studies are generally seen as small-scale versions or trial runs of the major study to test its feasibility (Polit and Hungler, 1987). Treece and Treece (1986) identified two purposes of pilot studies: (1) to make improvements in the research project, and (2) to detect problems that must be solved before the major study is attempted. The value of pilot work can be seen in the possibility of occurring serendipity. Not all weaknesses can be detected because a pilot study is artificial and the sample small.

It is impossible to pilot interviews exactly as each is a unique encounter between researcher and subject. A trial run, however, can help to detect, for example, the interviewee's general understanding of the topic and the questions, any inconsistencies within the interview guide, a researcher who is talking more than the subject, and many more aspects.

The first two patients were selected for a trial interview where practical and technical matters were tested. These pilot interviews were satisfactory, the responses entered the main collection as rich data emerged.

Main study

After successfully conducting two pilot interviews, another 18 patients were interviewed using the semi-structured interview guide. The talks took place either in the patient's room if he/she was alone or in a quiet room on the ward.

The interviews were recorded with a tape recorder because it is most probable that writing down notes during an interview means that a long period of time would be spent on writing, the interviewee might forget something through the interruption, eye-contact would be lost, certainly nonverbal cues overlooked, and errors might occur when answers are scribbled down in a hurry.

The analysis of phenomenological data

The goal of phenomenological analysis is the interpretation of data with faithfulness to the phenomena (Knaak, 1984). It is a rigorous process of intuiting, analysing, and describing the tacit and explicit meaning of experiences presented by subjects (Parse et al., 1985), the three operations were originally defined by Spiegelberg (1982). 'Its purpose is to derive from the collection of protocols, with their naive descriptions of specific examples of the experience under consideration, a description of the essential features of that experience' (Polkinghorne, 1989:50). There is, however, not one method but many, depending on the phenomenon under study and the aims of the researcher (Colaizzi, 1978; Riemen, 1986).

Well-known methods are, for example, those developed by van Kaam (1959, 1969), Giorgi (1975), Colaizzi (1978), Spiegelberg (1982), and Hycner (1985). The methods differ in elaboration and in the sequence of the single steps, but their common elements are always bracketing, defining of meaning units, determination of common themes, and description.

Wertz (1983) emphasized the importance of the comparison of individual descriptions in order to gain a wider understanding and to see an individual's experience from a different point of view reflecting past descriptions. Fischer's (1971) description of a structure of privacy is an example for this approach. There exist different views on the feature of the description of phenomena. Colaizzi (1978) pleaded for an unequivocal description without transformation of the meaning. Reinharz (1983), on the contrary, pointed out that there are automatically five steps of phenomenological transformation. The first is the transformation of an experience into language, the second is the transformation of what the researcher hears into understanding. Thirdly, the researcher transforms this understanding into clarifying conceptual categories. Without this step 'one is simply recording, and recording is not enough to produce understanding' (p.79). In a fourth step, these categories are transformed into a written document, and in a fifth step the researcher's audience has to transform the written word into understanding. It is important to bear in mind that during all those transformations something can be lost. This is of particular relevance in the present study, where the original language has to be translated at one point

41

of the analysis, a procedure which in any case distorts the original meaning to a certain degree.

The method of analysis employed in this study is mainly based on an adaptation of Giorgi's (1975) and Hycner's (1985) approach. It was argued that the direct application of one prescribed method would be rather restricting and, therefore, not suitable for the phenomenon under investigation. Thus the method used draws on aspects of both these authorities' recommendations.

Stages of phenomenological analysis

1 *Verbatim transcripts.* After recording the interviews, great value was set on transcribing them on the same day. One reason is the number of interviews to be conducted, another more important reason is the assumption that the memories of the interview are still in the mind of the investigator (Hutchinson and Wilson, 1992). For this purpose a Personal Computer was provided by one of the hospital staff where the researcher could install her own word processing program. A wide margin on the typed transcripts allowed notes on the same page. The interview guide then represented the top sheet of the transcriptions to facilitate easy orientation (Schatzman and Strauss, 1973). A complete copy of all transcripts was kept safely at a remote location in case of any mishap.

2 *Bracketing.* From now on the difficult procedure of bracketing was employed. There is not one single step of bracketing but the phenomenological reduction is performed throughout the whole analysis. The researcher tried to free herself of any concepts or presuppositions concerning the topic to let the data speak for themselves.

3 *Identification of meaning units.* The researcher listened to the tape and read the transcripts several times to get the sense of the whole interview. This provided the background and context for identification of the meaning units. Meaning units are those 'words, phrases... which express a unique and coherent meaning (irrespective of the research question) clearly differentiated from that which precedes and follows' (Hycner, 1985:282). The original interviews being in German, it was felt that as the literal expression had to be transformed into a meaning unit anyway, this was the most suitable time to do the translation, an approach that differs from Giorgi's (personal correspondence) who advocates the translation of the transcripts. However, it seemed to the author that a translation at this stage would distort the meaning least as meaning units are more comprehensive than verbatim transcripts.

4 *Checking of each meaning unit for relevance to the research topic.* In this stage each single meaning unit was examined to see whether it answered the research question or not, i.e. if it reflected the interviewee's experience on privacy. If in

doubt whether a unit fulfils this requirement, it is generally better to include it than to lose data that might have proved important at a later stage. This applies especially to all those pieces of information that made sense in the interview but seem impossible to code during the analysis. The determined units were phrased in the third person and put in numerical order to facilitate location.

5 *Clustering the meaning units under a common theme.* During this stage an effort was made to identify common features among the remaining meaning units. This was done by rigorous interrogation of the meaning of each individual unit by bracketing and entering the participant's life-world. To validate this step, it is useful to go back to the transcripts for a safety check to make sure that no meaning is lost during the previous stages (Colaizzi, 1978). This usually very time consuming and labour intensive stage can be performed much more comfortably with a good word-processing program. There was, however, the problem that the researcher had to cluster English meaning units with the German verbatim expressions still fresh in mind, which proved to be a very strenuous task.

6 *Independent judges.* Normally one would ask at this point independent referees to verify the findings. As there was no time for analysis in Germany it was not possible to use independent judges for the analysis of the data because of the original language of the interviews.

7 *Identification of general themes.* All clusters of meaning units were again examined to determine the presence of central themes.

8 *Identification of general and unique themes for all interviews.* After the analysis of all interviews up to stage seven, themes that were common to most or all of the interviews were identified. This is a difficult task because one has to determine the common meaning on one side but also has to accept individual differences. Themes that are unique or appear only in a few interviews were determined as well. Finally the transcripts were read again to make sure that no evidence was overlooked.

Salsberry (1989) in her critique of the phenomenological method claimed that searching for common themes is contradictory to the aim of the method, namely uncovering the unique experience of the individual. One must, however, argue that the mere determination of themes that occur in a great number of subjects does not diminish the importance of the unique experience.

9 *Writing a summary.* On the basis of step eight a summary was produced that describes accurately how the phenomenon under study is experienced by the interviewees (see Chapter 3). The results could then be compared with available

findings of previous studies on the topic. In this last stage theory development occurs that is based on the findings of the investigation (see Chapter 8).

Summary

After the determination of the research aim and the objectives, the research setting was described. A short introduction to the philosophy of phenomenology as well as the justification of the use of the phenomenological method in this present study was provided. The development of the interview guide and the way of sampling was explained. The ethical aspects were considered and the data collection was described. The analysis of the data was structured in nine steps, the findings will be presented in the next chapter.

3 Patients' perceptions of privacy (1)

In this chapter the findings of the patient interviews are presented. The interview guide provided a general structure for this presentation, additional themes which emerged during the analysis were integrated. The following categories demonstrate patients' concerns about their privacy while in an acute care setting:

- Privacy in general
- Privacy in the hospital environment in contrast to home
- Fear of exposure of personal identity
- Personal autonomy
- Fear of physical exposure of body
- Territoriality
- Personal space
- Intimate distance
- Effect of invasion of privacy on the individual
- The individual as part of a patient community
- Coping mechanisms/reactions to invasion of privacy
- Features of the hospital experience that should be changed

Several times categories overlap but it was the aim to describe experience as recounted by the informants, the idea of splitting themes in order to categorize them was found to be impractical and was, therefore, at times abandoned.

All evidence is identified with a number which refers to the patient (see Table 3.1); evidence without codes always refers to the last mentioned patient. Verbatim quotations will allow the data to speak for themselves and so illustrate the description. The author's comments are in square brackets.

Table 3.1
List of interviewed patients

Pat	Sex	Age	Ward	Length of stay	No. of beds	Mobile	Bld.
01	male	53	surgical	5 days	4	yes	new
02	female	72	medical	5 days	2	yes	new
03	male	70	medical	7 days	3	yes	old
04	female	61	medical	3 days	4	yes	new
05	male	21	surgical	6 weeks	4	part.	old
06	male	46	medical	4 days	2	yes	old
07	male	41	surgical	4 days	2	yes	new
08	female	80	surgical	5 months	2	part.	new
09	male	83	surgical	4 weeks	2	yes	new
10	male	51	medical	3 days	4	yes	new
11	male	80	medical	6 days	2	no	old
12	female	71	surgical	4 days	2	part.	new
13	female	31	surgical	4 days	2	yes	new
14	female	46	oncology	4 days	3+1	yes	old
15	male	80	surgical	38 days	2	no	old
16	female	27	surgical	10 days	1	part.	old
17	male	51	surgical	26 days	1	no	old
18	female	33	medical	7 days	2	yes	new
19	male	67	surgical	5 days	1	yes	new
20	female	79	oncology	18 days	2	no	old

Privacy in general

At the beginning of the interviews the patients were asked what they understood by the term 'privacy'. Apart from one patient who was not sure at this stage (10) three themes emerged: Protection from body exposure, data protection/confidentiality, autonomy.

Protection from body exposure
Privacy is being alone during personal hygiene procedures (1).

Data protection
Confidentiality of data was the main concern of one lady (2) and a gentleman (6) who had already had a bad experience was very sensitive about disclosing information about himself, 'I don't feel always happy when I have to fill a questionnaire and have to tick which institutions may have my data... It is like with the bank, you don't know exactly who has access.'

46

Autonomy
The majority of the responses could be attributed to this category. 'To do what one wants (5)'; 'free to do what one wants (19)'; 'to be independent and to be able to do what I want (11)'; 'to do things one never would do in public, one closes one's door and is within one's own four walls (17)'; and 'to make one's own decisions (7)' were the answers. For a couple, their home represented privacy (8; 9).

Privacy in the hospital environment in contrast to home

On this topic more patients had comments to make. This resulted in a variety of answers. Many of these themes will be presented in more detail as they were explored at certain stages in the interview guide. They are mentioned here only when the patient named them to illustrate what he/she meant by the difference between privacy in hospital or at home.

Not much difference from home
There was not much difference between hospital and home, as he had everything he needed (1).

There is a big difference from home
Home and hospital are like day and night (17). For an elderly lady (20) it was a big adjustment to go to hospital as it was for an old gentleman: 'In the hospital I lose my privacy. This is very important. It is difficult to leave my home at my age [80 years]... (11).'

There is a difference in sanitary facilities
The sanitary facilities were, of course, different from those at home (13).

Data protection
The difference starts when one enters the hospital (14). Unfortunately, personal information must be accessible to many people in hospital (2). One patient (6) feared that his right to confidentiality was jeopardized in hospital.

Autonomy
Although generally happy with his stay in hospital, one patient (1) did not like not being able to get up and get something to eat when he felt hungry as he could do at home, he reassured the researcher that 'generally, nobody has to be hungry here.' He didn't like the food. One patient (6) missed certain conveniences like his music instruments or his language course. One lady (20) reported: 'They put me in a room, told me to get undressed and go to bed.'

Everybody knows that hospital is different from home
It is clear that a hospital is not like home. If one has too many expectations one is only disappointed (4). On admission to hospital the differences from home are noted and institutional rules must be observed (7). One lady (12) agreed with this patient.

Hospital is like prison
Surprisingly, two female patients came up with the analogy of the hospital being like a prison. One lady referred to the spreading of information among patients (14), the other said: 'I told a girl friend, here it is like in a prison [laughs], everything is controlled (16)', referring to the accessibility of her belongings.

Patients are accessible at all times
A problem in hospital is that patients never can be alone if they wish. One patient (10) suffered because it was not possible to be on his own. 'In hospital anybody can come in at any time (5).'

Free from family for some time
A young lady (16) with a big household who stayed in a single room saw the difference from home in a positive light. Although there were a number of problems with her privacy in hospital, being away from her family for a while was a nice change.

Would rather stay at home and suffer more
Although he was very satisfied with the atmosphere in hospital, one patient (3) missed his home environment and stated:

> I would rather suffer more if I could stay at home. I wouldn't mind to suffer more and get the medical treatment I have here at home. I would prefer that. I have a very harmonious family life, I would say this is the best treatment for me. When I am at home I know how the day will be, I am sure that nothing bad happens and I am content. I like this safety...

The specified details that make privacy in hospital so different from home are described in the following sections.

Fear of exposure of personal identity

In this section the patients were asked how they felt their identity was protected. The following aspects emerged:

- exposure to full view of strangers and probability of recognition
- patient's data at bed or door
- questioning and discussion of private matters in front of others
- privacy with visitors
- privacy at the telephone
- discretion about events connected with patients

Exposure to full view of strangers and probability of recognition

It is embarrassing to be recognized as a hospitalized patient. Admission to hospital was seen as a rather private event. Attempts were made to reduce the number of people who knew of this. Therefore, one patient (2) found it embarrassing to meet people from the same village or town. Another lady (14) hoped that the construction workers on the scaffolds who could see her through the window did not know her. The same patient said:

> The next embarrassment starts when you are transported in your bed for an investigation. I had a gastric tube which is not very decorative and was taken for a gastroscopy. For this you have to cross the entrance hall. There comes another nurse, they exchange a word or two, and you are completely helpless and in full view of everyone. This is so embarrassing and degrading. Especially in this area where everyone knows everyone. And they say, oh look, she is in hospital, she is so pale, she'll turn up her toes soon...

It is perceived as an insult to be exposed to the full view of strangers. But even without the threat of meeting familiar faces, the possibility of being watched by strangers was experienced as an insult. One patient (6) had to wait in his bed in the corridor for one and a half hours. Other patients' visitors were already coming and watching him which made him very angry.

Patients' data at bed or door
Apart from a small label on the bed of surgical patients to prevent their beds from being mixed up in the theatre, there was no identification of patients either at the door of the room or inside the room nor on charts at the end of the bed.

It is a minor issue if names or charts are accessible. Some patients did not mind at all if there were names and/or charts or not (8; 15). 'The layman doesn't understand it anyway' (7). Another patient (10) did not mind although it was no one's business that he was in hospital. An elderly gentleman (9) found being in hospital is human, he felt that any healthy person could be in hospital next week and have to go through all the same procedures, he, therefore, did not mind. One patient (3) referred to the war when it also did not matter if somebody could read one's name or not. He stated that certain diseases like a sexually transmitted disease would not be written on the charts anyway, and

> I don't mind if they know I'm in hospital. When you are a passionate walker and you don't turn up, people say: where is so-and-so, I didn't see him today?, then my wife tells them I'm in hospital… When I'm missing in the village, somebody knows I'm in hospital.

Names at the door would make it easier to find out who is in hospital. One lady found it rather a pity that there were no names at the door as she wanted to know who was in hospital (13), now she had to check at the inquiry desk. She did not mind her name or birthday disclosed nor her charts as people would not understand them anyway.

Concealed names are a sort of protection of privacy. The majority of patients did not feel comfortable at the thought of having names and charts disclosed to the public and appreciated the custom of concealing the patients' identity (1; 2; 6; 12; 16; 18). One patient (5) knew of charts at the end of beds only from cartoons and approved of the current system. Names at the bed just make people curious and he wouldn't like that, was one statement (19), 'a hospital is a very private and personal place.' Two patients argued that concealed data would prevent people from gossiping how ill others were and how long they might have to live (4; 11).

People can draw conclusions from the ward's speciality. One lady was glad that names and diagnoses were concealed (14) but from the type of ward she was on people could draw conclusions about her medical problem anyway.

Student nurses do not protect confidentiality. Another patient (17) who preferred that his identity be protected was, however, sure that student nurses did not care much about data protection and although they were obliged to do so they contravened the rules.

Questioning and discussion of private matters in front of others
Apart from the patient in a single room, all other patients have to face the fact that during ward rounds or other staff-patient communication situations the patient's case was discussed in front of others and questions had to be answered. As many aspects are rather personal, patients were asked how they felt about disclosing personal issues before an unauthorized audience.

It doesn't matter to talk about private things in public. Some patients did not at all mind speaking about personal things in public (3; 8; 11; 12). One elderly

50

gentleman (15) stated, 'I don't have an embarrassing disease. I have a heart disease or something like that. This is respectable [laughs].'

Everybody hears from each other, it levels out. Others found comfort in the fact that everybody had to face public interrogation and although personal things may have been the issue, it did not 'really' matter as it 'levelled out' (1; 9; 20). One patient (7) was initially puzzled that personal matters were so discussed but the second patient had the same problem, so he no longer worried. 'I don't mind if the nurses ask about my bowel movements because everybody is asked (5).' A lady stated:

> ...anyone who doesn't like that has to take a single room and pay for it, I think. I hear about other patients and they hear about me. In the end it doesn't matter. They hear my business and I hear theirs. One has to be tolerant. And who can't stand that has to get private insurance and take a single room. That's how I see it. (4)

Certain topics should not be discussed in public. There were a number of comments indicating that however liberal they might feel about discussing personal things in front of other patients there were certain criteria where this would not apply. Certain diseases, might they be embarrassing, serious or 'complicated' should not be discussed (1; 5; 15; 17). Specific examples were a miscarriage (16), a contagious disease, 'I would be afraid of being ostracized' (7), but also 'questions about my sex life' (19). One patient remembered an incident as insulting when he was asked if he had proper heating at home (6). 'I found that impertinent. It was a consultant and I was so puzzled that I asked him what exactly he meant.'

> Well, it depends on the topic. If, let's say, if these are more intimate things, the doctor should discuss these with the patient alone, because one doesn't know the other patients. Well, you might know them for a few days but you don't know if they talk about it. Even if they don't, it is my business. One can talk about having to go to X-ray but, well, if somebody needs a certain therapy or is an alcoholic it should be discussed in private. I would ask the doctors to discuss this in private. I am sure the doctors on this ward would do it. (18)

Personal matters must never be discussed in front of others. For some patients public questioning was of great concern and they agreed that personal issues should be discussed in the doctor's office. One elderly lady (2) did not want private information on her history and her feelings spread which, unfortunately, had to be done in hospital, 'otherwise the doctor doesn't get a picture of me. The doctor will probably get a picture much quicker than a nurse who just implements orders.' All her data were only her and her doctor's business, not the other patients'. 'Confidentiality is a farce when patients can hear what I have.' Examinations and history-taking should be done in the doctor's office which would not be expensive or more time consuming. She also felt so distracted during the ward rounds that she could not concentrate or forgot what she wanted to say. 'Many things seem not so important during the ward round.' She made, however, an exception when she felt that a nurse really wanted to help her. She did not mind then discussing private matters. One lady (14) found it very embarrassing to reveal personal data in front of others:

> After the admission the doctor has to complete the admission form and to ask questions in front of two or three patients. One talks in a low voice but it is embarrassing. My mother, for example, refused to talk about her private life in front of all patients … Sometimes the doctors don't think. There are only two doctor's offices on the ward which are usually occupied. I understand the problem but I don't accept the situation. It is embarrassing. Other patients listen if they want to or not. When one is in hospital one gets big ears. It is like in prison where the paroles go around immediately. This is terrible… It is nobody's business but it has to be [being questioned].

One patient (10) suggested that patients who could not walk should be transported in their bed to the doctor's office to have privacy. 'Some people might say they don't mind being questioned in front of others but it affects everybody. Some are not so sensitive but it affects everybody.' (16).

Other patients' cases are not of interest. Interest in other patients' cases was different. Some patients emphasized that they or the others would not listen (1), were not interested at all (12) or found it embarrassing to listen to others' discussions (15).

One cannot help overhearing conversations. One does not listen but cannot help overhearing discussions (5). 'You can't help but overhear the others' discussions. It has to be quiet in the room, otherwise the doctor can't hear. So I switch off the radio. You overhear the conversations if you want to or not.' (10)

Some people are curious. One patient claimed he would not listen but that there might well be curious people around (11), 'diseases are very interesting'.

Listening to discussions on patients' cases are strenuous for the patient concerned and the listener. Other patients tried not to listen to topics that might embarrass the other patient (1; 10) or that were frightening or disgusting. One lady (2) used her radio with earplugs to prevent her from overhearing her neighbour's conversation because she sympathized very much with this patient and found this stressful.

It is good to know other patients' cases to deal better with them. On the other hand, there were patients who liked to hear about other patients' cases in order to share their experience (9) or to get to know them better, to sympathize and to consider them more (19).

Patients should know each person on a doctor's round. Two other remarks about doctor's rounds shall be added here. One patient appreciated that the groups were small and he was generally asked if medical students might attend (6), another patient didn't like strangers in the group, 'if I don't know this person who watches and listens I feel disturbed because it could be anybody.' (5)

Privacy with visitors
Visiting hours are for most patients a welcome change in a hospital day. Apart from unscheduled visits from friends or relatives, visiting hours are often used to discuss private matters.

There are means to achieve some privacy with visitors. Only a few patients (15; 16; 19; 20) felt they had enough privacy with their visitors, one (12) had nothing private to talk about. One lady (4) had no problem as her visitors were 'so intelligent that they reacted to small cues', she disguised or adjourned talks or left the room. One gentleman did not mind discussing private matters with visitors as he had no grave secrets (9). If necessary he could phone where he could talk differently or he would use different wording or adjourn the talk. Three patients who had enough privacy recognized the fact that there would be no privacy in a bigger room (15), where it might be necessary to whisper or make signs and one may even have no privacy at the phone (19) or where she would have to leave the room because she would always have the feeling that others would listen (16).

One patient (11) only had privacy with his visitors when the second patient left the room. To whisper, to leave the room or to wait until discharge were the solutions some patients employed for talking with their visitors in private (6; 18). One patient adopted these solutions but found it troublesome (10). 'Especially family matters shouldn't be public', stated one patient who mainly left the room when he had to discuss private matters with his wife but also thought of whispering or phoning (3). He was sure that patients don't hear every word that is spoken. 'There is no privacy with visitors. They have to listen if they want or not, except everybody has visitors and they are busy with them (14).'

> One has not many private things to discuss but one has to whisper, you know, there are so many and you hear them even if you don't

want to but somehow you catch it. One could use the earphones and watch TV. I have to watch TV that I don't hear the others. Otherwise one would have to have a single room. But I'm not that sensitive. (13)

One lady pointed out that she did not hear or listen to what others discussed (4).

Bedbound patients do not have privacy with visitors. Bedbound patients, however, would have no privacy with visitors at all (1; 16) which would be very unpleasant (7).

There are not enough dayrooms. The lack of suitable dayrooms where patients could talk with visitors was criticized (1; 2; 18).

Other patients' visitors can be a nuisance. Other patients' visitors were sometimes seen as a major annoyance (7) especially if there are too many in a room that is too small anyway (15). One patient was disturbed by a fellow patient who was a teacher, who brought his work into the hospital and was visited by five or six colleagues every day (6). He was certain that this patient was very happy in contrast to him. Another lady (8) was not against visitors in general but she felt disturbed by other patients' visitors:

> There was an elderly woman from the Bavarian Forest who had many children and a lot of grand children, there was not a quiet moment from morning to night. It was very troublesome. I didn't complain but it gets on your nerves when you are ill yourself.

One lady (2) described her experience with visitors:

> The day before yesterday was my fellow patient's birthday and a lot of people visited her. Many people questioned her about her disease. I think it is not pleasant for this lady either, but unfortunately I can't leave the room. I remember a situation in another hospital which is still a trauma for me. There was a young farmer's wife who had an accident and who was well-known. Now, all the parish councillors came and whatever and she had at least 30 people who visited her, and continuously, I who was alone and had no visitors, continuously I had to listen to her history and how it happened. And when that happens 30-40 times a day, then, in fact you can't hear it any longer and you lose sympathy for this patient because you have heard it all too often.

Privacy at the telephone cannot be sustained

Even if some patients tried to use the phone to discuss private matters (3; 6) or to use it only for unimportant things (18) it was still a problem that other patients could listen, especially in larger rooms (19). She could say more at the phone in a low voice, one patient (14) stated, but there is only one phone per room and if more patients are bedbound one does not benefit a lot. 'Even nowadays the telephone in hospitals is still a luxury.' Although only in a two-bed room, one lady (2) did not feel at ease with phoning in front of somebody else as it involved much more:

> There is always somebody who listens, who also asks: who was that and such an expensive phone call from Düsseldorf and so long. She takes an interest and would probably feel funny if she didn't ask as she can hear me talking. This is very difficult. I try to explain that it was my daughter... and I also apologized that my grandson called at 9:30 pm, his parents are in Spain and he wanted to tell me that they know that I'm ill and all these things. And then I have a bad conscience because he called at that time... But I have to say something, what would she think otherwise? Maybe she would be unhappy because that may simply be her way. Maybe she is from a family where they talk about everything, you know...

Another patient (10) who was involuntarily in a four-bed room complained:

> Phoning is a big problem here. I have quite a lot to do in my business, big things are going on. You want to call and everybody listens. They even switch the TV off to listen better and afterwards they ask you what it was all about... When one can go to the public phone the problem is solved. If the phone is in the room it is the same as if you are talking to your visitors. When I get a call everybody listens. They don't know who is calling. Sometimes it is an important call and they wonder about my answers. There are some smart ones who ask then: what are you doing, man? what is in his head? ... In a two-bed room I could talk to the gentleman and ask him if he could leave for five minutes because I have an urgent phone call to make, I am sure he is understanding and leaves but you can't throw out three patients. Especially when one has drips and drains. One can't ask for that.

Discretion about events connected with patients

While walking in the corridor one patient (2) witnessed student nurses giggling and laughing about things they saw in a patient's room which she found very disturbing as it should not happen that patients witness something like that. She assumed this was a coping mechanism, 'they have to cope somehow when they get so stressed but Sister should tell them to do that in their rooms or in the nurses' office'. She felt the students might also laugh about her.

Personal autonomy

The themes which are described under this heading came entirely from the patients and were not part of the interview guide. It was decided to include this information because it revealed some of patients' concerns. The patients felt that autonomy, the possibility of making decisions concerning oneself, and to be taken seriously and respected as an individual also had to do with privacy.

Patients give up their personality and play their roles
One lady (2) found it amazing that one adapts immediately to the situation in hospital, gives up one's personality and plays patient. She played the same role she played six years ago. 'The patient surrenders and adapts.'

Patients are not respected as personalities
Nurses still call old patients Granny and Grandpa and say: now we do this and that (2). Nurses will never give that up. Another patient (6) felt that he was not taken seriously when he was left in his bed in the corridor for a long time and everybody stared at him.

A patient's daily routine is forced to change
She was forced to change her daily routine in hospital, one lady (2) said, as she was used to doing her literary work in the evenings.

Information in hospital is inadequate
Some patients felt they were not properly informed in hospital. Information was only provided if the patient requested it (2), and doctors should modify their language to enable the patient to follow the explanations, 'it has also to do with privacy to treat somebody as a mature person'. One elderly gentleman (15) missed being informed when nurses couldn't do certain things:

> The nurses are very nice when I need something but they don't tell you why they don't do something, they say nothing. I understand that they can't do everything because they don't have time. At the moment, I guess, the ward is pretty understaffed... but they don't say why they don't come. 'Yes, we are coming', but I can call half an hour later and she still didn't tell me why she didn't come. She can say why she can't come. The information is missing.

Staff consider personal preferences
One patient (14) appreciated very much that staff considered her wish not to be secured to the operating table before being anaesthetised because she panics in this situation.

There is no choice in meals
The same patient didn't like the fact that she could not choose and decide what to eat but had to accept someone else's choice, and she knew of many patients who felt the same way.

Other patients can force upon one unpleasant situations
One lady (2) was confronted with the situation that another patient whom she did not know took out her dentures and asked her to clean them for her. She felt awful but felt that she could not refuse and complied with the request. Another patient (3) was under considerable stress when he was confronted with suffering patients.

Suspicion towards hygiene in hospital
One lady (2) confessed she was extremely sensitive concerning hygiene:

> ...once I had a row with my husband because he stirred the food with the same spoon with which he had tasted it. My children said lately: 'how can you be so fussy'... And when you go with such an attitude into hospital... I still can get up and wipe the spoons although it is nonsense because I guess they are clean. I hope they are [laughs]... When they come with the washing bowl, you don't know if somebody... I thought, God, it looks as if there is still some soap at it. However ill I might be, I always see this because I'm so sensitive... I don't like it when the cleaner wipes everything with the same cloth. I told her that I would clean my bedside table myself. A tablet might be placed there by mistake or something I put into my mouth might touch the bedside table, I wouldn't want that.

Another patient (10) was concerned about the cleanliness of the bathtub and shower and demanded that a male nurse or a cleaner should make sure that they are cleaned properly after use [this patient felt that cleaning was the male nurses' job]. Other patients felt uncomfortable about leaving open food or drinks on the bedside table, especially over night, as one reads a lot about germs in hospitals (3) and one never knows if somebody touches it (14).

> I am concerned about the hygiene here, that's really the point, well, when I got the commode, the first thing I did was to clean it with disinfectant because I don't know who was sitting on it before. I know,

in all probability that it is only wiped with a wet cloth which is not enough for me. It wasn't dirty but the feeling somebody sat on it and it was only wiped with a wet cloth is revolting. (16)

Fear of physical exposure of body

In this section patients were asked how they felt their need to be suitably covered or screened at certain occasions was met. The emerging themes were as follows:
- Sanitary facilities provided in hospital
- Being washed
- Focus on treatment of intimate areas of the body
- Elimination
- Personal hygiene performed by nurses of the opposite sex
- Screens/curtains
- Opening doors without warning
- Wearing of operation gowns
- Doctors do not put themselves in the patient's shoes
- Active control over one's body

Sanitary facilities provided in hospital

Apart from patients in single rooms with an en suite toilet, patients normally have to share facilities either between the patients in a room with en suite bathrooms or between patients on the whole ward when facilities are located in the corridor. This sharing posed problems for a number of patients.

Sharing toilets does not matter. Two ladies in the new part of the hospital – one in a four-bed room, one in a two-bed room – did not mind the shared toilets (4; 13). The first one thought it would be too much to expect for every patient to have his/her own toilet, the second found sharing acceptable as they were only two in the room. Two gentlemen who had to use toilets on the corridor did not mind either (6; 3),

> …each cubicle is screened. There is one room with three toilets each of which is screened in a cubicle. There is no reason to bother. Maybe older people might mind noise or smell but I never bothered.

It is awkward to share toilets/bathrooms. Other patients were not happy to use toilets or bathrooms used by others (9). It was mainly a matter of hygiene which was seen as insufficient given the kind of patients one was confronted with. One lady (2) found it rather awful to share the toilet. Up to that point she had got up and disinfected the toilet. 'I find it stressful to use the toilet and to know the stoma patient was here earlier.' She assumed that the other lady did also not feel comfortable about this situation herself.

The four-bed rooms in the new part of the hospital had two en suite facilities. One patient did not like that as 'there is a coming and going, one uses one time this toilet, next time the other (10)'. He felt he had no control over who uses which toilet and found it unhygienic. He, therefore, escaped this conflict by using the visitor's toilet. 'They are really clean. I walk around until I find one because they are clean and cool and fresh.' Another lady (18) had the problem of sharing the facilities with a patient who, she assumed, was not very clean. She could use the shower only after the cleaner came because the other patient threw scraps of paper everywhere and the shower was full of it. Before that she had an old lady in her room who was messy but couldn't help it. So she took a cloth and cleaned the toilet. She did that but found it very unpleasant. An elderly lady (8) who now had an en suite toilet remembered the times when she had to use toilets on the corridor. People smoked there and she found it disgusting and she was always afraid to use those toilets.

The washing facilities are insufficient. To have only a wash-basin in the room was a concern for the patients in the old part of the hospital. Either it was too narrow to get there with the commode (11), the curtains were not adequate to feel properly screened (5) or washing at the wash-basin itself did not satisfy his hygienic needs (17). One patient (3) suspected that the wash-basin was not clean and suggested that every patient had to scrub it after use. He would like his own wash-basin for which he would be responsible. Now he is the first in the morning to wash when he is careful to inspect the wash-basin thoroughly. 'Hygiene is no luxury', as he emphasized.

En suite facilities are preferred. One reason why patients preferred en suite bathrooms was the long distance they sometimes had to walk to the toilets on the corridor (2; 5; 8; 18). The latter patient saw the distance as a major problem for surgical patients after operations or with crutches. For another patient (15), not having en suite facilities posed a complex problem. He could not get to the toilets as they were too far and he needed help every step of the way. He found the toilets the worst thing on the wards as they were too narrow to get into with a commode and there were also not enough toilets for the whole ward. He also did not have his own commode because there was only one with wheels which he needed as he had to be pushed to several places. An en suite bathroom would allow him to get there on the commode, there also would be enough space. He claimed that nowadays en suite bathrooms are an absolute must. 'Who would stay today in a hotel without an attached bathroom?'.

Patients who were lucky enough to be in the new building and to use en suite facilities complained about several imperfections concerning their privacy. Due to a technical fault the toilets were not soundproof and lacked sufficient ventilation. The whole room smelled after the toilet was used and both problems were very unpleasant (7). One patient (10) felt very uncomfortable about the possibility someone could hear him in the toilet. Another lady (18) had the same problems:

> ...it is dreadful that the toilets are not soundproof and have this bad ventilation. I think it doesn't work at all. The whole room smells. The smell goes into the whole room. It is very unpleasant if you have a patient in your room who doesn't like to open the window. It is very embarrassing when there are visitors. And you can hear everything. I simply let the water run [laughs]. One can keep the water running in order to subdue noises.

Generally, however, patients preferred the modern facilities in the new part of the hospital.

Being washed

To ensure personal cleanliness is an action that most people prefer to do in private. In hospital, however, patients can be dependent on the help of others and a private action becomes a rather public event.

Being washed is not important. There were some patients who did not mind being washed by a nurse or washing themselves in the room in their bed (6; 15; 19). One lady (18) did not mind generally apart from one embarrassing incident when she was a patient in the Intensive Care Unit and a young man who offered voluntary services had to wash her. She had had her menstrual period and he had had to remove a tampon.

It is unpleasant to be washed by a stranger. It was embarrassing for quite a number of patients to be washed by someone else (1; 2; 3; 5; 13; 14; 16). Before her operation it was of great concern to a lady (13) that she would be able to wash herself. Other patients thought although it is unpleasant one gets used to it after a while (10; 20). The first of those two patients put the blame for his indifference on the many drugs he had received. One patient (17) solved the tricky problem in that he let the nurses wash the 'normal' parts whereas he, his son or a friend washed 'the rest'.

Focus on treatment of intimate areas of the body

To be washed in intimate areas is an unpleasant event (3). An old gentleman (15) agreed and he wanted these 'embarrassing tasks' like washing, pre-operative shaving or having a catheter passed at least done by a male nurse. The sheer idea of having a catheter passed or any treatment in intimate areas struck one lady (13) with terror and she felt she would run away. One patient had had (7) several years earlier an unpleasant experience when he needed a coloscopy and he was not told that there would be a larger audience, probably students who wanted to see the investigation. The examination started when suddenly many people appeared. He was screened but the intention of the screen was that he didn't see the spectators. He noticed that this was done with almost every patient and found it very disturbing. But being embarrassed through treatment in intimate areas is an issue only initially, later one gets used to it. A lady (4) said that she has a big problem when anything has to be done in this area, be it a bedpan, a rectal thermometer, or gynaecological or rectal examination. She tried to place confidence in the person performing this and claimed that it would be a misplaced modesty if, for example, a disease is overlooked because she feels ashamed. The care of her colostomy was of concern to an elderly woman (20) who tried to handle it on her own whenever possible. To get a pre-op shave was no problem for one patient (19) but he put himself in the nurse's position and thought it must be rather unpleasant for a young female nurse to shave a man.

Elimination

Hospitalization means for many patients that the privacy in which body functions are normally performed can no longer be taken for granted. Various reasons can force the patient to use devices like urine bottles, bedpans or commodes and his elimination suddenly becomes an issue for strangers. The need to give in to invasion of privacy in connection with elimination was of serious concern to all patients. Some had already had some experience, others were frightened of ever finding themselves in this situation.

It is extremely embarrassing to use a bedpan or commode. After his operation a young man (5) had to use a bedpan and commode. He was visually screened as he sat behind the curtain around the wash-basin, but he found it very unpleasant because the smell bothered the other patients in the room. He is no prude but these are very personal things, said one patient (6) and referred to his absolute dislike of bedpan or commode. He had to use both once, the bedpan with a screen, the commode without. 'Very unpleasant' was how two patients described the situation (8; 9), the second added that there is no difference in embarrassment between a bedpan or a commode. However, he always imagines that somebody else might also need the bedpan. He has to tolerate it and he expects the same from others. Even for him as a former doctor is it embarrassing to use the commode which unfortunately he has to, because one bothers the other patients (11). To be smelled by others was also a major obstacle for one lady (12). She would leave the room if another patient had to use the commode

61

and she would not be happy if she was to become bedbound. An old gentleman (15) was, especially at the beginning, very embarrassed to use the commode in front of others. Urine bottles can be disguised in contrast to smelly commodes.

> The next embarrassment is when you had an operation and you are told to use bedpan or commode. Now, you are with three or four patients in one room. They are all women but I think... In former times there was a screen which was easy to handle. Everybody in the room knew what happened behind it but one had at least some feeling of privacy. But now one sits like on display. Have you ever tried to wipe your bottom in front of other people? It is dreadful. It is one of the most embarrassing situations one can imagine. Patients are forced to do this, where else should they go? ... It is difficult to ask visitors to leave the room if one of three or four patients needs the bedpan. It is embarrassing when there are visitors and I have to go to the loo. I have to call the nurse to tell her that I need the bedpan, then the nurse has to ask the people to leave, you know how it is... And I am the cause of all this fuss. Then the next point, you don't just pee into the bedpan but you use it also for 'big' business and the windows have to be opened [before the visitors enter again], believe me, this is terrible, this is terrible. This is very, very terrible. (14)

Although in a single room a young lady (16) who had to use the commode felt she had no privacy at all as there was no space behind the curtain at the wash-basin to position the commode. The idea of using the commode in front of others seemed dreadful to her. The fact of using the commode is bad enough but she assumed it might be easier with a screen. 'The sight is unpleasant.' She felt awkward when she was washing or sitting on the toilet and especially if strangers were watching her.

One patient (7) recalled that years ago after a car accident he had to use the bedpan which was very awkward. He was not allowed to leave the bed but he got up secretly in the night. He was sure that many patients got up secretly to avoid the use of the bedpan. He did not know how he would feel about it now but he assumed that he would not mind so much if his neighbour were in the same situation, even without a screen. The most awful situation, however, would be if the same happened with visitors. Not just the exposure but the smell, even of something so natural, was what he dreaded most.

Using a bedpan or commode was also very embarrassing for another lady (18) who would avoid it if at all possible. In case, she would prefer a commode because bedpans are freezing cold, cause pain and one never knew if the bed stayed clean. 'Some people are so inhibited that their bladder simply closes.' Although covered with the quilt one is not better disguised using a bedpan as everybody knows at the end when it is removed.

62

One gentleman (17) in a single room suffered terribly when he had to use a bedpan – the worst thing that could happen to him in hospital – and he said he could not stand to use it if other patients were in the room. However, he would not be bothered if somebody else had to use it.

One lady (13) reported that she simply could not use a bedpan. She did not know exactly what the problem was but she had inhibitions. She remembered that once she was supposed to use the bedpan but she could not. 'I thought my bladder would rupture, and in the end the nurse gave in and took me to the loo.'

Although not being a prude, one patient (19) admitted that there is one thing that really concerned him. He found it very degrading to use a bedpan to open his bowels:

> This is the worst thing that could happen to me in hospital. This is the worst. I don't know, perhaps I am a prude. I think, oh God, now the nurse has to… it is, I can't really explain how it feels. Well, I feel,… I think the whole day about it, God… This is so bad that it doesn't even matter if a male or a female nurse attends me.

One patient (10) had to use a bedpan in ICU a long time ago. He remembered that he felt very bad. He would not know what to do if he needed one now. He thought he would not be able to stand it. 'Either they have to keep me somewhere alone or they have to invent something. They have to find some other way or it is impossible.' Another problem for him was the mere sight of a commode in the room. He would complain immediately, 'either they have to take me out or they remove that patient or anything, but I can't stand it'.

One lady (4) agreed that using a bedpan or commode is very embarrassing but as everybody knows it is embarrassing, one can overcome this problem by suitable behaviour. She excused herself in advance for any inconvenience, they all laughed about it and understood and that was it. The next time somebody else had the courage and in the end it was no problem at all.

At the beginning, her colostomy was dreadful for one old lady (20). She found it disgusting but forced herself to care for it on her own. Now she had become accustomed to it and did not even mind if a male nurse cleaned it.

It is embarrassing to expose the contents of drainage bags. Catheters and drains are normally connected to a collecting bag. The content of those bags is visible to anybody. This was a problem, especially when she had to walk in the corridor with a lot of strangers around (14):

> I am so ashamed, I am so ashamed. People can see what is in the bags. This is something I can't handle well. When visitors come, I cover those things while they are hanging from the bed frame with a big towel. Above I talk, and underneath I don't know when something

runs into the bag, I can't feel it. It is also embarrassing for the visitor who doesn't know where to look, nor do I. It is unpleasant for me and I know it is unpleasant for many.

Personal hygiene performed by nurses of the opposite sex

It was assumed that some patients would have problems if more personal tasks were performed by nurses of the opposite sex.

There is no difference between male and female nurses. A number of patients stated that it would not make any difference at all if they were, for example, washed by a nurse of the opposite sex (1; 3; 5; 6; 7; 9; 10; 15; 18). One older lady (12) was never washed by a male nurse but she assumed that male nurses 'are used to this' and, therefore, she would probably not mind. Being washed by females was no problem anyway as all women look the same. Another old lady (2) thought these old ideas have to be overcome. 'One goes also to the male doctor or the masseur, when people are trained, sex does not make any difference.' One gentleman (15) was astonished how the young girls dealt with this, 'an old man is not a pretty man. But who cares?' and he was sure that the female nurses were very neutral. Another patient (19) said that female nurses do not mind seeing naked men and male nurses naked women because it is their job, therefore, he did not mind at all. A female nurse chose this job and it is part of it to see naked men or to touch them while washing. An elderly lady (8) had to be washed once by a male nurse. At first she was very reluctant but it turned out to be very 'natural, easy and non-stressful'. After that experience she would not mind at all. She was once washed by a diaconess/nurse who undressed her completely and washed her from head to toe. That was really embarrassing.

Preference of nurses of one's own gender. Other patients preferred to be washed by a nurse of the same sex (11; 13; 20). 'I would rather be washed by a male nurse although female nurses wash with more feeling (17).' Another lady (14) still preferred female nurses although she had met some male nurses who, in a particularly embarrassing situation, were very considerate and helpful.

> I am not modest but I trust a female nurse more. There is always some inhibition to overcome. Some say they don't care but they do. (4)

It was entirely out of the question for a young patient (16) to be washed by a male nurse. It is embarrassing for young women but older women do not mind so much anymore. Although she did not mind being washed by a male nurse, if she needed assistance for elimination she would have preferred a female nurse (18). In contrast to the former patient, she thought that the older women get the more they prefer to be washed by females.

Patients were asked if they would like to be screened on certain occasions. The response here is divided into three sections: (1) screens are not necessary, (2) screens are essential, and because patients seemed to distinguish between 'serious' invasion of privacy and less serious forms in connection with investigations or dressings, (3) screening for examinations or dressings.

Screens are not necessary. Few patients stated that curtains or screens between beds are unnecessary (4; 8; 9; 12). He might have wanted a screen in former times, an elderly patient stated, but he had overcome this feeling long ago and now he thinks screens are not necessary (17). The fact that in one room all patients are either male or female made a screen redundant (11; 17).

Screens are essential. There should generally be screens between the beds which could be used during many procedures such as washing, elimination, in order simply to have some peace behind it or in order not to be forced to watch very sick patients (2; 14; 18; 20). The fact that they were all women did not mean that it was all right being exposed (14). This lady was quite sure that patients do not really watch but the possibility and uncertainty of being watched is so unpleasant.

That one should be screened during washing was the demand of several patients (1; 3; 10; 16). One lady (4) who also thought one has to be screened for washing found it unpleasant when others had a wash and did not care to close the curtain. One patient (6) did not want to wash 'certain body areas' in front of others, especially strangers, and said a screen is absolutely necessary. Simply standing naked in front of somebody is not that embarrassing like standing naked in front of the wash-basin for a wash (16). It would be nice to have a screen for any intimate treatment (15).

Elimination was another occasion when patients wanted to be screened (8; 18; 19). But it would balance out as he could watch other patients in return.

ICU and admission wards were repeatedly named as examples in which patients had no privacy at all (18). When she was in ICU, there was a male patient next to her completely uncovered – probably because of all the machines – which she found very disturbing, and she suggested staff should think if this is really necessary (14). Another patient (10) had a similar experience when he was in an ICU where they actually had screens between the beds. Staff often forgot to pull them. Next to him was a young woman with exposed breasts. He told staff to draw the curtain and from then on they took care.

Screening for examination or dressing. Some patients emphasized the need for being screened for examinations or dressings (10). One lady (2) said it is very embarrassing, especially when somebody has a 'delicate' disease and needs dressing [referring to her neighbour who had a colostomy]. One patient (1) didn't want to be watched in 'complicated' areas, 'it is not very pleasant if there is a problem with your bottom and everybody watches'. 'Nobody cares if others are watching when my big abdominal wound is dressed (14).' Another lady (13) wanted a screen because 'one always has a look, even if one does not watch all the time [laughs]'.

A number of patients did not mind being watched on these occasions (1; 8; 9; 11; 15) as everybody sees everybody, it levels out (4) or because one gets used to it after so many times (5; 12). 'The others don't look different, maybe they have a little more or a little less (18).' This woman had the experience that women watch each other's body shape whereas men are in this respect not that complicated. A screen is not necessary because patients do not watch (6) as one cannot see so far (1). One patient (3) did not mind being watched but he did not want to see others suffer.

Getting undressed in front of strangers. Two patients did not mind getting undressed (7; 12), for others it was a major problem. One lady (18) changed her clothes always in the bathroom. One gentleman (17) reported:

> The problem starts when I have to get undressed. These are things I don't like, especially in front of somebody I don't know. It wouldn't be that bad with friends. I have no inhibitions with my wife or son. I slowly got used to nurses and doctors. It is better when I know them for a while. Now, if I had to get undressed in front of you [researcher] I would do that with a certain… mmm… well, let's say with certain inhibitions… I never could go to a nudist beach. This is something I couldn't do. I could run around naked when I'm alone but in Sylt or wherever, I couldn't… Maybe if somebody offers millions, that you say, well, do it once, but it is against my Catholic upbringing…

A young lady (16) had a wound at her chest and she had to undress to let the doctor see the site:

> That alone is enough. I'm not what you call prude but it is after all in front of complete strangers. I can't imagine anybody likes that… In the meantime I was three times at the X-ray department and each time you have to get undressed and there is always the doctor and three or four other people. This is embarrassing. I feel so exposed to them. It feels awful when there are three people who have practically nothing to do with you, they stand there, you have to undress and plant yourself in front of the machine. I feel uncomfortable. They see that everyday and I'm sure they don't watch me but they check the film or the position. They don't stare at my breasts but I perceive it like that.'

Patients have a right to watch. An interesting idea concerning being watched came from the same young woman (16). She thought patients watch in any case if they have the chance. It is boring in hospital, so people talk to each other and after a while they think they know each other quite well, which gives them the right to have a look.

Opening doors without warning

The patients were asked how they felt when somebody burst into the room while they were in a rather unpresentable state. Some patients did not mind when nurses burst in when not properly dressed (4) or standing naked in front of the wash-basin (1; 19). Nurses sometimes open the bathroom door to check a patient, but she would mind if strangers burst into the bathroom (13). One patient (10) thought he would be startled for a moment if he was undressed and the bathroom door opened but he wouldn't mind so much because one has to expect this in hospital. It would only be a nurse anyway. Other patients took bursting in more seriously. It is embarrassing to use the urine bottle and people suddenly open the door and have a look (17) or to have a wash and somebody bursts into the room whoever it may be (18).

The possibility of the door being opened is dreadful. A young lady (16) found it very annoying when the door opens during washing. When the door opens and it is busy in the corridor, anybody might have a quick look which is always embarrassing. The possibility of being watched is awkward.

> The visitor who enters the room doesn't know somebody is sitting on the commode. He knocks and opens the door. He closes it immediately but it is already too late. The simple possibility of somebody opening the door is dreadful. (14)

The same lady illustrated her opinion in another example:

> ...I had to get an enema which is usually done in bed. Impossible, I said, if the door opens I will have a heart attack. I told her [the nurse] I can't stay in the room, I don't mind lying on the floor, only, I don't want the door to open...

The nurse took her then to another room.

Wearing of operation gowns

A few patients did not mind wearing these, either it was only for a short period or they managed to keep them closed (1; 5; 6; 18). One lady (20) preferred one for of practical reasons as she could handle her colostomy better.

Other patients (9; 11; 12; 15; 16) found it very unpleasant to wear something that leaves the back uncovered, 'in the front cloth – at the back nothing' (8). One lady (13) thought they should have at least a button but then her neighbour reassured her that they look all the same. One patient (7) did not mind if patients saw him but he would not want visitors to see him in an operation gown. Another gentleman (3) found it disturbing that people walked around in operation gowns, 'a man doesn't look very becoming when you can see him from behind', and he thought that nowadays everybody could afford proper clothing. He would not walk around like this, he would feel very irritated. Two patients said they would discreetly look away if they saw a patient in an operation gown (8; 9).

Doctors do not put themselves in the patient's shoes

One patient (14) had to have a sigmoidoscopy which is in itself an unpleasant examination. She found it embarrassing to lie there as the doctor examined her:

> ...the door opened and in came another doctor. He said hello, you say hello as you are a polite person, and the doctor goes on with his examination. Doctors tolerate this, I don't. You know, one is so exposed... but you can't do anything. That needn't be. He examines your bottom and says to his colleague, Sir, do you know this or that... or you talk and he removes polyps or whatever. It feels so strange... The position is so degrading.

Active control over one's body

The presentation of her body was of great concern for a lady (14). Patients who come from recovery room are generally still sleepy. It happened once in a train that a passenger opposite her fell asleep. 'Do you know what a face he pulled? And this is exactly how you look like when you come from the theatre and are in your room. One is in full view of everyone'. She explained that she does not like to be watched in her sleep because she feels defenceless. She can defend and control herself when her eyes are open. It is unpleasant not to be in control in front of strangers.

Territoriality

Bearing in mind the literature on the functions of territoriality and an individual's reaction to invasion, it was important to explore patients' perceptions about this topic in a place where they have to establish their own territory anew and defend it against repeated invasion. The following themes emerged:

- What belongs to patients' territory
- Room size is important for well-being
- Additional bed
- Knocking
- Personal belongings have to be moved for cleaning
- Available space for toilet articles
- Accessibility of belongings
- Reasonable safety of belongings
- Opening of bedside table or wardrobe
- Sitting on the bed
- Leaving items on the bed
- Changes in the environment/removal of furniture
- Moving rooms
- Staff using the patient's telephone

What belongs to patients' territory
The patients laid claim to different sizes of territory. After having the questions explained, one patient (3) reassured the researcher that he would not want to claim one square metre, all he wanted was a place near the window because he needed a lot of oxygen in his condition. The bed was a lady's (2) only territory as she was the only occupant whereas the bedside table or wardrobe were accessible to anybody. Bed plus bedside table was named three times (5; 6; 14), the last patient deplored the lack of a wardrobe of her own. Other combinations were: bedside table, space around the bed, wardrobe (1); bed, bedside table, wardrobe, shelf for toilet requisites (4); bed, bedside table, half the table (8); bed, bedside table, wardrobe, the right to use the toilet (12), this lady stressed she would not want to claim half of the room. Other patients did claim one half of the room (13); half the room, half the table, the crucifix and the window (11) or:

> ...my area is the bed, bedside table, wardrobe. I expect that a certain area is seen as mine and respected. I also expect that the sitting area at the windows is divided. I wouldn't claim the other half but I expect the same for my half. The empty space is divided equally and it has to be accepted without discussions... For the meals the table is strictly divided into two halves. (7)

A fixed place at the table was also important for other patients (18; 15), 'the same place at the table feels a bit like home'. One patient (10) saw a certain space around his bed as his territory but couldn't specify it.

One lady (14) criticized the fact that when patients have to stay for a long time or until they die, there was no possibility to arrange the environment to give it a more personal touch.

Preferred room size. Patients were asked what room size they would prefer if they could choose. Quite a number of patients would have preferred a single room (11; 16; 18; 19). Unfortunately they were too expensive (2) or there was no single room vacant (6). His big problem and only reason for choosing a single room were snoring fellow patients. Two ladies wanted one or, at the most, two beds in a room (13; 14).

Two-bed rooms were also a desirable arrangement. In older hospitals, two-bed rooms are reserved for private patients, this was the reason why two patients referred to money when they answered (4; 15), others knew that newer hospitals had two-bed rooms as a standard (7; 8; 9; 10; 20).

A four-bed room was preferred by two patients because they liked the company and there was a bit of entertainment (1; 12). For one patient (5) the room size was irrelevant.

Less favoured room size. Some patients did not like single rooms because they were bad for very ill, bedbound patients (7; 15), they were boring (12) or made one feel lonely (20).

Four-bed rooms were also not much liked by some patients (15) because there was always noise and trouble (10) or because they were felt to be dreadful (18). Although there might be some fun, one patient (19) would have preferred not to try. One lady (16) did not want anything larger than a single room.

Additional bed
In times of overcrowding there is sometimes the need to place an additional bed in a room.

It is bad to get an additional bed. Additional beds were not liked (1; 8; 9). 'There is no space and no oxygen left (3)', 'no space left (18)'. One lady (14) who had a fourth bed in her room wished that it was not there.

One has to tolerate an additional bed

> Once I had to tolerate an additional bed which I didn't like. I had a single room and they told me, somebody else had to come because there was no space. Well, what could I do? Of course, he needs a place, so, come in. But I didn't like it. (6)

Another lady (12) was in the same situation having to accept an additional bed. There was not much space left for her but 'one mustn't be so choosy'. An additional bed would bother her because of lack of space and she would not like it but you cannot do anything about it (13). One patient (19) would tolerate it for a short period such as one day, otherwise he would not agree and would react accordingly.

It is embarrassing to be the additional patient. He had to be an additional patient once, said one informant (6), which was not pleasant. He was very grateful to his 'host' who agreed to the arrangement as he was supposed to stay only for a short while. In the beginning he assumed that this patient was angry but it turned out that he was very nice. The embarrassing thing was that he didn't know how long he would have to bother this gentleman.

A patient (10) who was at the beginning of his stay in hospital as the fifth in his four-bed room told of his experience:

> I was the fifth and in the middle of the room, this is very annoying...
> Well, there were already four in the room, you know. I came as the
> fifth, that was strange. You lie in the middle of the room. It wasn't for
> long, maybe half a day. Nobody could enter the room, the male nurse
> couldn't pass, nobody could pass my bed properly, it is also for them a
> hindrance. And you are watched from all sides, everybody looks at you
> and watches your movements.

Knocking

A person who enters another person's room enters his territory. To make the owner of the territory aware of the imminent invasion it is customary to knock on the door which represents the territory's border. The question was if people who enter a patient's temporary territory do the same and how their action was perceived by the patient.

People knock. Some patients reported that people mainly knock (1; 3; 5; 7; 8; 9; 11; 12; 13; 15; 17; 20). Two patients stressed that visitors knocked before entering (4; 10). It has to be pointed out that some of these patients were private patients who seemed to get 'privileged' treatment.

Not everybody knocks on the door. Of the staff only some nurses habitually knock, the others simply burst in (3; 4; 6; 10). One lady (2) who made the same observation said she is certain it depends on the staff's upbringing whether they knock or not.

Prefers knocking. Some patients definitely would appreciate it if staff knocked before entering (2; 6; 11). One lady (20) wanted to be warned before the door opened and a private patient (19) wished that everybody would knock but he did not like it when doctors did not wait for an answer before entering. One lady (13) said knocking did not bother her as it is not loud and she knows when somebody is about to enter the room.

71

Student nurses should learn to knock. Although he did not mind if people knocked or not, one patient (17) wanted the students in the nursing school to be told to knock. When nobody knocks, the students do not learn to do so (2).

Knocking is disturbing. One lady found knocking disturbing (4) and one gentleman had not considered if he minded knocking or not as he had more important things to think of (10).

Knocking has no effect. Doctors and nurses knock and open the door immediately, said one patient (14), she did not mind whether they knocked or not but she saw it as pointless. A young lady (16) said:

> ...the nurses knock once and they open the door. The door is open at the same time... They knock so fast that I can't say: a moment, please. They open the door and you sit there [on the commode]... The annoying fact is: knock and open. It is not a question: may I come in? but more a: hello, here I am. If they didn't knock, the noise of the opening door would have the same effect. It goes: knock and open. I have no chance to answer.

Another lady (18) had the same complaints with doctors:

> They knock and are in the room straight away, they don't wait for an answer. Pressing the handle has the same effect. Knocking is sheer politeness but has no effect.

One cannot expect nurses to knock and to wait for an answer. Nurses cannot wait until somebody bothers to answer (14).

> I understand that there is not much time and they can't wait for everybody's response. Many patients are very ill or sleep or watch TV or don't hear well, the nurses can't wait. (16)

Another lady (18) said that she did not blame the nurses when they did not knock because sometimes they were carrying a tray or a syringe.

Did not like the door slamming or being left open. The door's function as a territorial border was the concern of one patient (6) who hated it when nurses slammed the door or left it open. 'They say they are coming back and then they leave the door open.'

Personal belongings have to be moved for cleaning

Most people did not mind when somebody took their personal belongings away to clean the bedside table (1; 6; 7; 8; 9; 11; 12; 14; 15; 16; 18; 19). It would be unfair to expect a clean bedside table and complain when somebody touches these items (4). Another lady (13) took those items off herself so that the cleaner would not be bothered. 'One mustn't be so sensitive (20).'

Although he did not mind generally, one patient (5) did not want his radio touched (5), another patient (10) insisted that the cleaner ask before removing anything.

Available space for toilet articles

It was assumed that sufficient space for toilet requisites was seen as necessary, i.e. that articles are not too close to and mixed up with those of other patients.

There is enough space. Depending on their room design, some patients said that they had enough space for their requisites (1; 2; 3; 5; 7; 18). One lady (20) in a two-bed room in the old building was satisfied with the space, she emphasized, however, that four-bed rooms provided the same space and then it would not be enough. One gentleman (6) had enough space because they were only two in a three-bed room.

Not enough space. Others felt that they did not have enough space to store their toilet requisites (14; 15; 16). 'It must be terrible to share this little space with more patients in a larger room.'

Storage of towels. One patient (12) was glad that towels could be kept separate from those of other patients. Others were not happy that there was not enough space to keep them apart from other patients' or to have the possibility to let wet towels dry properly because of lack of hooks and racks (3; 6; 15).

Accessibility of belongings

Quite a number of patients felt uncomfortable at the thought that somebody might use their toilet articles or towels, especially when they had en suite facilities where they had no visual control over their belongings (11; 12; 13; 18). One elderly lady (2) was concerned when her neighbour's visitors used the en suite toilet, she was not sure if they used her towel [laughed]. She didn't trust these simple people to have good manners. To prevent this situation, one lady (18) demanded that visitors must not use patients' en suite facilities. One lady (16) did not like having her toilet articles displayed and in full view. She found it very unpleasant when the cleaner took her things and scrutinized them. Everybody knew which cream she used.

Three patients wanted to be on the safe side and took their requisites back after use. One patient (14) did not think anybody would use her things but she did not want to leave them in the bath, especially not her toothbrush and paste. She always put them back in a bag and back in the room although this was not ideal. Another patient (18) did not want others to look at or use her toilet articles. One gentleman (10) had already had a bad experience:

> Today one asked me: whose towel is this? I said: it is mine. He had it already in his hands. The problem starts already there. You can't even leave a towel there [en suite bathroom], you can't leave anything. You have to take everything back to your bed or lock it in your bedside locker. Such are the problems. Everybody has his own towel or one from the hospital. But you are not there to watch what they are doing.'

Reasonable safety of belongings

Patients felt generally that their belongings in the bedside locker or in the wardrobe were kept safe (6; 13; 15; 19). Wardrobes could be locked but they left them open, because he had nothing valuable (1), because there is always somebody in the room (2), because he trusts that nobody would take anything (6), because there were nothing but clothes and he expected that his property would be respected (7). A fellow patient (20) had taken one lady's purse by mistake, apart from that incident she felt that her belongings were safe.

Only one patient (10) was not satisfied with the safety of his property. Especially for valuables he wanted a safe in the wall as he had had in another hospital.

Opening of bedside table or wardrobe

Patients were very firm in their view that nurses should not open the bedside locker or wardrobe without permission (6; 10; 11; 13; 16; 19; 20). Nurses might open the wardrobe as there are only clothes but not the bedside table (18). One patient (15) could not see his wardrobe and hoped that nobody opened it. Other patients mitigated this view and said they would not mind a nurse opening their wardrobes if they were very ill or in case of an emergency (1; 3; 4). One patient (9) said, it would only be in his own interest if a nurse opened wardrobe or bedside table, he, therefore, excused this behaviour.

Sitting on the bed

As most patients felt that their bed was their territory, the researcher wanted to know how they felt about people occupying this territory by sitting on the bed.

People may sit on the bed. Two patients did not mind others sitting on their beds (11; 16). The second patient felt she had no special relationship with her bed at all. Other patients agreed to it when there were many visitors and they had nowhere to sit (10; 15).

Did not like people sitting on bed. Some patients disapproved of the custom of people sitting on patients' beds (1; 8; 9). Two patients substantiated their rejection with hygienic reasons, 'maybe he had just come from the street or had used the tram (2)' or 'one never knows what sort of disease a person has' (12).

Family may sit on the bed, strangers may not. There was a general notion that family members and close friends could be allowed to sit on one's bed. Strangers such as other patients, visitors or staff, however, were not allowed this privilege (4; 5; 14). One patient (10) whose friends were well-mannered enough not to sit on beds said he did not want staff or doctors on his bed because they take his space and his feet hurt. One lady (13) once made an exception for a nice lady doctor. Another patient (6) who did not like strangers on his bed assumed that staff might have reasons to sit there. If nurses sit on his bed, at least they had to talk to him and not to anyone else in the room (7). One patient (19) distinguished between familiar and unfamiliar nurses. If a nurse whom he did not know well sat on his bed it would look 'as if she wanted some sort of contact.' Doctors were allowed to sit on his bed. One lady (20) tolerated her family for a short while on her bed, another patient (3) saw fellow patients as his friends which gave them the right to sit on his bed. One lady's family did not sit on beds but she would not mind a nurse doing so (18).

Leaving items on the bed
His own visitors' coats may be laid on his bed, a patient said (7). Others did not like this (1), mainly because it was unhygienic (3; 12). A nursing tray could be left on his bed (3). If it was a tray with nursing material for another patient, he would tolerate it only for a short while (5). One patient (10) did not allow anything on his bed:

> ...if a nurse leaves a tray on my bed I would complain immediately. I would throw it down automatically by kicking it with my feet which is easily done. It never happened but I would tell her to remove it because I don't like this.

Changes in the environment/removal of furniture
A certain set of furniture or equipment can be expected as part of a patient's room. Sometimes it is necessary for nurses to 'borrow' a chair, an arm-chair, a wheel chair or whatever to use it in another room.

Patients did not mind too much (1) if not too many pieces were taken (3) and if they are brought back clean (4), which certainly would be done as she trusted the hospital.

One lady (12) did not mind if the windows were opened without asking her permission as she liked them open anyway. One gentleman (11) wanted to be asked. A bedbound patient would certainly be disadvantaged if a nurse opened the window without asking and there was nobody to close it for him (1).

Moving rooms

Sometimes it happens that patients have to be moved from one room to another for organizational reasons.

Patients who were moved said it is always difficult to readjust each time (14). There is always the uncertainty of who the next set of patients would be (5). One patient (7) wondered where he would be taken to. He was moved into a room of the same design, however, he had to adjust to a very ill neighbour.

Staff using the patient's telephone

Patients could rent a telephone for the duration of their stay. These phones could also be used for internal calls.

> I don't like this business with the phone. Anyone can come in, doctor or staff, take the phone and make a call. I assume that these are internal calls that don't cost anything. But it is annoying. I don't like it when a doctor comes in and makes a call. It is not the point if it is charged. The point is that he has nothing to do with my phone. I pay 2 DM per day for it. (10)

Personal space

Considering the importance of personal space in our interaction with other individuals, patients were asked how it felt when other people or when nursing or medical equipment were positioned close to them.

Distance from individual to people or equipment

Beds are positioned close. Other patients could be disgusting, therefore, he liked some space between beds (5). Another gentleman (10) agreed and demanded there should be more space around the beds. One lady (14) did not mind if another patient was close.

Equipment is positioned close. When patients were asked how they felt about drip stands or nebulizers for other patients being positioned close to their beds, two did not bother (1), as it is necessary for this patient (14). One gentleman did not like it (5), another found it always annoying (10), a third did not want someone else's drip stand in his area or even see another patient's monitoring machines (6).

Strangers stay close to the bed. Visitors of other patients must not sit close to him (10). One lady (14) did not like when strangers leaned at her bed:

> ...it drives me up the wall. The bed is shaking. It doesn't hurt but I don't like it. It is my bed. He is invading my area [...]. I don't like anybody leaning on my bed. I don't like anybody leaning on my car. I don't do it to others and I expect the same, especially regarding my bed.

Another patient (18) did not mind others leaning on her bed but she did not like people standing close and watching every movement.

Patients standing at the window. It was assumed that patients whose bed stood close to the window did not like other patients standing there. Two ladies did not mind at all (14; 18). One gentleman (11) would tolerate it only for a short while. Another patient (6) whose bed was far away from the window stated, the window is everybody's territory. There might be people, he said, who feel annoyed about it.

Patients have to pass the bed closely. Patients whose beds were close to the mainly fitted wardrobes were in the situation that other patients had to pass sometimes very close to reach their wardrobe.

It does not matter, said two of the informants (1; 4). 'You cannot do anything about it anyway' (12). One lady (13) said, one has to accept it even if you do not like the other person. One patient (6) who was not close to a wardrobe but to the wash-basin did not mind his fellow patient standing close to the bed while washing, he simply turned away.

Intimate distance
Due to its nature, nursing involves a great deal of touching of the patient. With regard to Hall's intimate distance (0-45 cm), this touch could be interpreted by patients as an intrusion of this intimate space.

One lady could not comment as she had not been touched up to that point (13). Others did not mind at all (5; 8; 9; 11; 15), 'as long as it helps' (3) and if it is necessary, not as, for example, if she had to get out of bed and a male nurse grabbed her although she could have managed alone (16). One male patient (7) did not mind being touched as long as it is not in a peculiar way. Another gentleman (6) was sure that nurses do not touch deliberately, 'they are sometimes in a hurry and lean over the bed instead of going around.' If anybody took his hand during a conversation, it would very much depend on the topic if he is annoyed or not. 'One can't help being touched when bedbound' stated one patient (10), and he assumed that the sicker one was the less one cared if it is unpleasant. One lady (4), however, did not like being touched at all.

It does not make any difference who invades one's privacy. Three patients reported that it does not make any difference who invaded their privacy, it was always an unpleasant experience (4; 14; 16).

Dependence on others. Dependence on others, patients and mainly nurses, was a topic of concern for some patients. Patients depend on nurses who help them with things they would normally do themselves (5). It was especially embarrassing, when nurses have to assist during or after elimination. 'It was very embarrassing, the nurses had to come five times an hour' (6). '... and the nurses have so much work and have to run and carry it [container of commode] away' (12). Another patient (19) found the dependence on nurses who have to empty his bedpan or commode excruciating. Depending on others for minor things was also a problem:

> ...it is embarrassing to be so dependent and have to call ... When it is dark and the light is on I can't use the commode but I have to call for somebody to close the curtains. One is terribly dependent. (16)

One elderly gentleman (15) was embarrassed when he had to call out for somebody. He didn't like to be dependent because he had no control over when this person would arrive.

One could also feel dependent on another patient. One informant (6) who had to stay as an additional patient in a single room felt himself to be at the mercy of his 'host' and did not know how long he would have to bother him.

Did not like to be helped. One gentleman (17) generally did not like being pampered. He especially dreaded assistance in using the bedpan. As soon as he could get up he moved around in a wheelchair which exhausted him terribly, yet it was better than having to ask someone for help:

> I don't mind if somebody else needs a bedpan. I am a person who would rather help somebody than be helped. If the phone is out of reach I would ask somebody to get it for me, that is a small matter. But I don't like to ask for help with personal things.

One has to be grateful for help. Even if being washed by a stranger felt awkward, assistance and help during those times when the patient was not able to perform this task for himself was gratefully acknowledged (3; 5; 6; 9; 14; 19). Interestingly, this gratitude focused solely on being washed.

One has to give in. Patients felt they were at the receiving end of the hierarchy of power, and how ever much they resented certain things, in the end they had to concede and accept whatever awful or embarrassing events they might be subjected to. One had to accept being washed (1; 18) or – awful though it is – to use bedpan or commode (7; 13; 17). One patient (6) surrendered for his own benefit and gave in to giving personal data, using a bedpan/commode or accepting an additional bed. Another patient (7) stated, one has to overcome inhibitions in order to get help, he even tolerated students watching him during an embarrassing investigation because he thought everybody has to learn sometime. One gentleman (15) had to accept using a bedpan/commode, being catheterized and to being unscreened during examinations.

Patients are forced to do degrading things one never would do in public (14). As a patient, one has to give in to everything that is connected with a stay in hospital (19). One elderly gentleman (9) felt one cannot do anything, one is in the hands of doctors and nurses, he quickly added that he meant this in a good sense. He surrendered to the service and received the service in return, it is based on mutual trust. Trust was also the basis on which another patient surrendered more easily (3).

In illness modesty and embarrassment are abolished. From a certain severity of illness on it appeared that any obligations to appropriate behaviour are abandoned. 'Fact is, when you are ill, it doesn't matter who has a look, one overcomes that' (1). 'One swallows a lot when one is seriously ill, you wouldn't do it if you were healthy, but it has to be' (3). One lady (4) stated, the sicker one is the less one cares who examines…, when one is sick one makes concessions and is not difficult about it…, and many things are acceptable when one is very ill. 'The sicker someone is the less one bothers' (5). One lady (14) felt:

> You lose any modesty after a while. But not with civilians. The difficulty starts with student nurses, it costs me an effort, but how much more in front of strangers… After an operation one doesn't mind much being washed by a stranger… When I am very ill I don't mind being touched.

One gentleman (9) said he makes concessions because he needs the help. The question is of essential tasks he could not do himself and he needed the others and their altruism. One lady (20) got so used to constant invasion of privacy that she did not mind anymore, 'you become cold.'

The individual as part of a patient community

Expected behaviour of people
Patients expected fellow patients respect each others' privacy and behave accordingly. 'People don't watch' (1), 'I don't think that they really watch' (2), 'If she is

a decent person she doesn't look' (4), 'people don't watch, even at delicate sites' (6), 'patients don't hear every word' (3), and 'people don't listen' (4) were common answers. The informants did not do certain things and expected the same in return regarding, for example, using somebody else's towel (19) or watching others (8; 14).

> If another patient's privacy is invaded I studiously don't watch, one looks away. If I don't watch I expect the same from others... If I met my neighbour after some time I wouldn't use the information I have about her and I expect the same in return... This is something about trust. (4)

One patient (7) expected tolerance and understanding and he also expected people to behave accordingly.

It is a matter of manners
People's behaviour is a matter of manners or upbringing (2), 'there is a certain etiquette' (9). There are, however, people who do not know how to behave. 'One simply can't expect it from some people, it is beyond their capabilities. I would feel sorry for this person, not angry' (8), not everybody behaves accordingly (9), some people have no manners (14). When a patient is examined, she (18) leaves the room. Some patients stay out of curiosity, some are polite and leave, 'it is a matter of manners.'

Relationship between patients
A lot depends on a good relationship between patients (2), 'another patient would have said: take a single room.' Harmony among the patients in one room is important and improves recovery (3; 19). One lady always (8) experienced nice and understanding patients. Another lady's (4) need for privacy depended very much on how she got on with the others. If she got on well she became more open. Privacy might not be such a big problem when the patients get on well (7). As the other patient was very nice, he (6) did not feel so bad when he had to occupy some space in a single room. Privacy could be a major problem if there are unpleasant patients who do not get on well (13), if there was someone she did not get on well with she would be ashamed. This person could say at home that she is fat. When the relationship is good, it is good to share the experience and discuss personal matter and give advice. It happened to him (9) that one patient wanted sympathy by telling him everything. Both were ill, shared suffering calls for openness. One lady (20) had a bad experience in a four-bed room when one patient demanded that she be removed from the room because of her colostomy. She felt it was not her fault and the incident shocked her terribly. Luckily she gets on well with her current neighbour.

80

One has to consider others. Sharing the same fate with others calls for mutual consideration. Respecting others' needs was seen as important (3; 5; 7; 13). One has to consider others' needs even if she is disadvantaged, for example, she wouldn't open the window if there was a patient with pneumonia, she would get fresh air outside (4). There are, however, also inconsiderate and reckless people around (4; 5). An eccentric fellow who always wanted his way was not appreciated (3).

Conformity among patients. A big problem in rooms with more than one patient was that there had to be a certain conformity concerning issues which affected everyone. The example which was cited most often was the opening of the windows. Many people like fresh air in their rooms (3; 18) and suffer if not all the patients agree to keep the windows open or at least open them regularly (2).

> It is bad when somebody doesn't open the windows. That is the problem. I love fresh air, many love fresh air, but there are also many who keep the window sealed and that's unbearable. It is difficult to find a solution with many patients. I can give in with certain things I don't like but I can't live without fresh air. If I feel cold I can cover myself, but the air, terrible, terrible. Just enter a room with a patient who doesn't like to open the window, dreadful... One has to act in conformity with the others. She is right who shouts loudest. (14)

Matching suitable patients. To ensure a fairly problem-free stay in hospital, patients should be matched to fit together. One lady (4) wished that moderately ill and seriously ill patients would not be together in one room as it is very stressful to be confronted with severe illness. One patient (10) was angry that staff who knew about his business and that he had to phone a lot, put him in a four-bed room where he was constantly bothered by the others, instead of asking if he preferred a two-bed room. One lady (18) wanted the patients to be of about the same age, 'I can't get better when I have to share a room with four grannies [laughs].' Older people need more warmth, younger people want to keep the windows open. Young and old shouldn't be mixed.

Coping mechanisms/reaction to invasion of privacy

Reaction to problems

One patient (7) did not know how he would react, others' reactions were varied. Two patients would solve the problem by not making a big fuss but trying to move to another room (3; 5). One gentleman thought (6) his reaction probably depended on the event and the person. He would be stricter with patients than with nurses. In other things like opening the window he would try to find a solution or surrender angrily.

Other patients stated that they would not complain (8). In the case of being questioned in front of others, she (16) would not complain because she could not imagine that doctors would be able to consider this factor out of time constraint. In one incident, a patient (4) did not complain because she did not want to give offence. It is a matter of upbringing how these things are dealt with. If things get worse she covers herself and hides in her snail-shell, her bed. She does not maintain contact to people who do not respect her privacy. Another lady (14) also felt she wanted to cover her face when she was transported through the entrance hall or close her eyes.

However, if it gets too much, she would complain (4). 'When it is too much, I would politely say something' (18). One lady (2) had major problems with her neighbour who wanted the window kept closed. She had to assert herself when she opened the windows. She started to lie and say the window is closed but in fact she drew the curtain so that this patient could not see the open window.

> One has to protect oneself. One can change behaviour in an assertive way. I was brought up to behave in such a way as not to harm anybody. If somebody does something because she is malicious or ignorant I would say something. I would explain why I have to open the window. This is the way to do it. (4)

One lady (14) employed a very sharp angry glare to make clear that something was amiss. Some people, however, did not get the message, then she felt like leaving. Another lady had a lot of problems with a patient who did not open the windows. 'It was terribly hot, I couldn't sleep and it stank'. She discharged herself from hospital against medical advice (18).

Patients don't complain

He never heard any fellow patient complaining about invasion of privacy (5). Patients' opinion is never sought and they are afraid to say anything (17). One lady wondered why patients do not complain if they do not like something but put up with everything (14).

Features of the hospital experience that should be changed

At the end of the interviews patients were asked what they would like to change if they could. Although the interviews were full of data, at this stage only a few patients wanted to comment. It appeared as if the hospital as a complex organization with its regulations and its traditions could not be expected to be concerned with this sort of complaint. If they said anything, 'I wouldn't know what' (8; 12; 15; 19) was the answer, or 'there are always improvements possible, but I wouldn't know what' (9).

The toilet facilities were mentioned by two patients (7; 10), the second wanted his own toilet, knowing that it was rarely feasible.

Better manners were desired by one gentleman (11), a smoother organization by another (6) and a no-smoking policy in the hospital:

> I would stop smoking in the entrance hall, it is an affront. One opens the hospital door and out comes smoke. It is a catastrophe. It is very bad, I would suppress it. A hospital is not a smoking-room. One has to be strict. Not just because somebody can be harmed but also as a health educational issue.

A proper receptacle for toilet requisites would be reasonable (16) but the most passionate demands were made for proper screens (14; 16).

Summary

The results of the patients' interviews have been presented. A variety of themes emerged from the vast amount of rich data, illustrating how patients perceived privacy in hospital and of how much concern certain issues were. The findings show no major surprises or contradictions to the general theories of privacy and territoriality. Intrusions into personal space seem to have less effect on the patients than might have been expected. Whether it is in itself less relevant or whether this aspect is simply overshadowed by the evidence about exposure of identity or (to an even greater extent) physical exposure, cannot be extrapolated from the present set of questions asked of the patients. The findings represented the basis for developing the second stage of the research in which a Likert-Scale questionnaire was employed to examine how topics under consideration are perceived in a larger population. It might be expected that those results will not differ greatly from the interview findings. The methodological aspects of the second stage of this study are discussed in the following chapter.

4 Method 2 – questionnaires

Design of the study – second stage: questionnaires

Based on the findings of the interviews described in the previous chapter, it was planned to examine if similar trends could be found using a larger sample. This chapter describes the methodology of the second stage of the data collection. It starts with a discussion of the advantages of triangulation. The justification of the chosen approach is outlined, the stages of the development of the instrument are described, and the method of analysis is discussed.

The quantitative research
Quantitative research methods count or measure. They present their findings in terms of numbers, frequencies, amounts (Hockey, 1991). The aim is to produce quantifiable data amenable to statistical comparisons.

Application of different research approaches
Frequently the qualitative and the quantitative approach are combined in one study. This combination is often called 'triangulation'. Denzin (1978) differentiated between data, investigator, theory, and methodological triangulation. Burgess (1984) used the term 'multiple strategies'.

Data gathered by different methods can be seen as more valid and reliable than others gained by a single method, because the limitations and weaknesses of one method can be at least partially counterbalanced by others (Denzin, 1978; Jick, 1979; Pan American Health Organization, 1983). This is seen to increase the comprehensiveness of the study (Goodwin and Goodwin, 1984). But it does not mean that mistakes made in one method are balanced by a correct application of the other (Fielding and Fielding, 1986). However, one can assume that validity increases with the use of triangulation (Brink, 1991).

Jick (1979) suggested that qualitative and quantitative methods should be seen 'as complementary rather than as rival camps'. He defined some advantages of triangulation: Firstly, researchers can be more confident of their results. Secondly, divergent results can lead to enriched explanation of the topic. Thirdly, the use of different methods can lead to a synthesis or integration of theories, and finally, triangulation can function as a critical test for competing theories.

When it is under consideration whether to triangulate or not, an attempt has to be made to balance efficiency and adequacy of methods against constraints like time and available resources (Duffy, 1987). In this study triangulation of different methods was used to examine if the data gained through interviews from a relatively small sample are supported on a larger scale. On the basis of the interview findings, a Likert scale type questionnaire was developed to investigate the degree to which a larger sample of patients agreed with the emerged themes. Oppenheim (1992) amongst others (for example Price and Barrell, 1980) suggested this kind of procedure. The advantage is that qualitative data can be used to generate hypotheses which are then tested quantitatively.

The measurement of attitudes
An attitude has been defined by Oppenheim (1992) as a 'state of readiness, a tendency to respond in a certain manner when confronted with certain stimuli' (p.174). It is 'reinforced by belief (the cognitive component) and often attracts strong feelings (the emotional component) that will lead to particular forms of behaviour (the action tendency component)' (p.175). Attitude measurement is based on the assumption that individual attitudes can be ranged according to underlying dimensions (Moser and Kalton, 1971). A general limitation of measuring attitudes was seen in the fact that it is based on self-report which relies on the individual's knowledge about his attitude (Nunnally, 1978). A number of well-known attitude measuring scales have been developed in the past. One of those is the Likert scale which was employed in this study.

Likert scale
The Likert scale was originally designed to measure attitudes towards race relations, international relations, and economic conflict (Likert, 1932). It is a compilation of a number of statements. The informant has to indicate the degree to which he shares a viewpoint expressed in the statements (Polit and Hungler, 1987; McLaughlin and Marascuilo, 1990). As the respondent places himself on a continuum, no independent judges are necessary for this task (Bond, 1974). Mainly psychological traits are represented by a total score that identifies the informant's place on a continuum from positive to negative. In this study, however, it was not the total score of the respondents that was of interest but the sample population's rating of single items that emerged from the interviews. The topic of the present questionnaire is 'privacy'. It consists,

however, of different areas such as fear of physical exposure or territoriality. A patient who might be very sensitive in the first area might be very careless in the second. Therefore, most considerations regarding the original Likert scale do not always apply here.

Construction of items/statements. Constructing items for attitude scales is a difficult task. When – as in the present study – the scale is based on findings of a previous stage and especially on interview findings, it is very useful to select the wording of the statements from the interview tapes (Moser and Kalton, 1971; Oppenheim, 1992). Most important is the use of opinions not facts (Moser and Kalton, 1971; Smith, 1981). Neutral or extreme items make the data meaningless. Only favourable or unfavourable statements should be used (Nunnally, 1978; Kidder and Judd, 1986; Sommer and Sommer, 1991). An approximately equal number of positive and negative statements make the respondents read each item carefully and prevent them from producing a biased score (Nieswiadomy, 1987). The items have to fulfil many requirements, they should be exciting to the respondent (Oppenheim, 1992) and not biased or ambiguous (Barker, 1991). Edwards (1957) compiled a list of suggestions that help to construct usable items which were used as a guide in the present study.

Item analysis. The analysis of the single statements is most important in the development of a scale. A group of people are asked to answer the question-naire. Nunnally (1978) suggested the number of subjects should be no more than ten times the number of items, McDowell and Newell (1987) accepted five times as sufficient. The correlation of the response to each item with the total score has to be calculated (Kidder and Judd, 1986). Items that do not correlate highly should be discarded. This method is called 'internal-consistency method of item-analysis' (Oppenheim, 1992) as no external criteria are available. The limited number of subjects and time constraints did not allow such an elaboration in this study. Consequently, the findings have to be seen as suggestive rather than as conclusive. Apart from that, as no summational score was sought, item-analysis was less relevant.

Scoring. The responses have to be scored to be analysable. The most common way of scoring the response is to allow the respondent to use one of five possible degrees of agreement (strongly agree, agree, uncertain, disagree, strongly disagree). In his famous *Survey of Opinions* Likert (1932) himself used this way of scoring and also the three-point scoring ('yes', '?', 'no'). If the subject is offered five possible answers, the positive items would yield the highest score (5) for 'strongly agree', the negative items for 'strongly disagree'. All items have the same mathematical weight (Sommer and Sommer, 1991). Interestingly, people seem to try to avoid extremes, a phenomenon called 'error of central tendency' (Moser and Kalton, 1971).

86

Several authors (Burns and Grove, 1987; Nieswiadomy, 1987; Polit and Hungler, 1987) dealt with the question of whether or not to include the intermediate response. The disadvantage is that it can discourage the respondent from taking sides, its advantage is to leave an option if one has no opinion on a particular item. If 'uncertain' is used very often, however, the data may become useless. If this response possibility is omitted, the respondent is forced to choose an answer that does not represent his view and he might refuse to answer at all. The intermediate response could, however, be excluded as long as it is clear to the respondent how to indicate non-response (Youngman, 1978). So, although the author wanted the patients to decide, the category 'uncertain' was included.

Validity and reliability. A questionnaire has to undergo tests to ensure a certain degree of validity and reliability. Reviewing literature on this topic, one is struck by the different and often controversial approaches. Youngman (1978), for example, stated

> Standard concepts of reliability and validity have limited relevance in questionnaire design. Validity is typically assessed in terms of face validity, more often than not a euphemism for doing nothing (p.26).

One has, therefore, to decide carefully which way of checking is suitable for the desired purpose.

It is essentially a matter of judgement whether or not a questionnaire is valid. Sommer and Sommer (1991) suggested checking the validity of a scale by testing it with subjects who are known to have strong opiniona – positive or negative – on the topic. There are, however, limitations as topics are often multidimensional, as in the present study. Slocumb and Cole (1991) developed an instrument to validate the content of items. It is argued that the questionnaire employed has content validity because it was built on previous research findings. Concurrent validity could not be established as there is no known instrument that measures privacy with which this questionnaire could be compared (Brink, 1991).

Reliability tests of questionnaires consist of test-retest checks, split-half checks and equivalent forms checks. Test-retest checks are easy to administer but certain problems have to be borne in mind: the tested characteristic must not have changed within the two applications, and the memory effect could make the check rather meaningless (Moser and Kalton, 1971; McDowell and Newell, 1987). Whatever check is employed, items that are responded to in the same way by all subjects are normally unsatisfactory and have to be discarded. However, in this study the summational score per respondent was not of interest but the attitude of the sample to each item. Therefore, such items remained in the pool.

Sampling
This second stage of the data collection took place on the same wards (surgical, medical, oncological) in the same hospital as the first stage (interviews) about

six months earlier. The hospital directorate was aware of the research plan and had expected the researcher.

The ethical aspects were considered equally for the second stage. Two hundred patients were included in the second stage of the data collection. The rationale for this number was that a number of 40 patients on each of the five wards should be a sufficient size to gain the opinion of a wide range of different people. An effort was made to represent both genders equally. It turned out that, like in the first stage, female patients were rather reluctant to participate and stated they would not want to risk saying anything negative about the hospital and the staff. The respondents had to be in a state that allowed them to comprehend the task and to fill the forms accordingly. Convenience sampling was employed. The procedure of obtaining a sampling frame from the wards to randomly select suitable patients seemed to be rather impractical and complicated and was not possible in the available time. Unusual hot weather during the time of the data collection made many prospective patients cancel their operation or hospital stay so that very ill patients were over represented who could not be approached. The Olympic games posed another problem as patients wanted to watch their favourite sport transmissions throughout the day. Depending on the situation in the research setting, the researcher was prepared to enlarge the sample which was, however, not necessary.

Self-completion of a questionnaire puts additional strains on hospitalized patients. They may feel unwell, for example, be in an uncomfortable position to write, get tired easily, or are frequently interrupted through ward activity (French, 1981). Bored patients, and those were mainly younger patients on the surgical wards, saw the questionnaire as a welcome change, some busy patients felt at first rather bothered.

Pilot study

Prescott and Soeken (1989) stressed that pilot studies also have other potentials, for example to answer methodological questions and to function as part of the development of a research plan: 'pilot work serves to guide the development of a research plan instead of being a test of the already developed plan' (p.60). This pilot study did not only test the use of the Likert scale as such but also if it is a suitable instrument to serve its purpose.

Development of the questionnaire

First stage

The questionnaire started with a short introduction and an example of an answered question. The next section consisted of biographic data which can be a good start for a questionnaire because they are easy to answer (Youngman,

1978). Sixty items were extracted from the original German interview findings, not from the translated results presented in Chapter 2. In this way, problems that usually occur when instruments have to be translated (Jones and Kay, 1992) could be avoided. The wording was checked by several German medical students on the campus. This test could only be done by Germans as they are familiar with the meaning of the statements because of the common cultural background. They also completed the questionnaires. These results were used to pilot coding and analysis before the actual data collection.

Only minor rephrasing was necessary. Some items were worded in colloquial German as obtained from the interviews. It seemed necessary to use a language that would suit everybody in the sample.

Second stage
The complete scale was taken to the setting in Germany. Staff of the hospital were asked to check the scale. Changes in the construction of the statements were not necessary.

Third stage
The complete scale was administered to a convenience sample of ten patients on the same wards where the interviews took place. They were observed for difficulties and for timing. Because of the high turn-over rates it was not possible to conduct a test-retest check with the same patients. The patients stated that especially the negative statements took all their concentration. Modifications and re-tests were not necessary.

Main study
The data collection took place on the same wards as the interviews to ensure that the patients came from the same environment. An information sheet for the patients was designed to introduce the study and to emphasize the voluntary nature of the participation and the confidentiality of the data. After thorough instructions the forms were personally distributed to each patient and checked for completeness when collected. Patients who wanted to participate but had difficulties in filling the forms were assisted, in such a way that they told their response to the researcher who then completed the form accordingly. Some bias triggered by the face to face encounter can be assumed in contrast to the patients who filled the forms in private. But in this way, a 100 per cent response rate was achieved.

On the last page of the questionnaire a ranking list with 12 items was attached. This part of the study is described in Chapter 6.

Analysis
A Likert scale is usually summational, i.e. the total score of a respondent is calculated. The disadvantage is that a total score might have little meaning as

different response patterns could add up to the same score (McLaughlin and Marascuilo, 1990). The response pattern might be of greater interest than the subject's total score (Oppenheim, 1992). In the present study, primarily the score per item was of interest, therefore, the items were analysed individually, and not added to a score for each patient.

Because of the great number of patients (n = 200), it was decided to analyse the data by computer. The coding of responses started as soon as the first questionnaires returned to save time, what Lofland and Lofland (1984) called 'productive analysis'. A coding list was prepared to determine which code numbers matched which item on the questionnaire. The codes were then transferred onto data sheets which facilitated easier entry of the data. The coding was checked for accuracy. There were no missing data. The data were processed with the SPSS/PC+ software package.

Statistical Package for Social Sciences (SPSS/PC+). SPSS/PC+ is a widely used program which facilitates a variety of data manipulation. One advantage is that it is easy to learn. Helpful textbooks are provided by Frude (1987), Norusis (1988) and Foster (1992). Collected data are converted into numerical codes. Data sheets are filled with these codes which enables an easier entry into the computer. After that, the desired data manipulation can take place using the appropriate commands.

The analysis consisted of
- sample characteristics; it was expected that there might be different findings regarding gender, age groups, length of stay, size of the room etc.
- frequency counts
- cross-tabulations of variables with Mann-Whitney-Test, Kruskal-Wallis-Test and Spearmen rank correlation coefficient as appropriate. These nonparametric tests are suitable for samples obtained through nonprobability sampling and for the nominal and ordinal data collected.

Summary

The development of an instrument for the measurement of attitudes is a rather difficult task. In this chapter, theoretical issues were outlined, the Likert scale was introduced and validity and reliability of scales discussed. Furthermore, the development of the questionnaire, its application in the setting and the analysis of the data was described. The results of this stage of the study are presented in the next chapter.

5 Patients' perceptions of privacy (2)

This chapter presents the data of the Likert-scale questionnaire. After the description of the biographical data, the scoring rates are summarized under the same themes as were the interview findings to facilitate an easier comparison. The data from the questionnaires were cross-tabulated with the variables sex, age, days of stay, number of beds in room, ward and building. In the following sections, differences between the sexes, the age groups, the length of stay, number of beds, the different wards and the old or new building are recorded. Correlations are only mentioned where significant.

Biographical data

Altogether 117 (58.5 per cent) male and 83 (41.5 per cent) female patients participated. The age range was from 17 to 87 years, divided into four age groups which seemed to represent best the different life-styles based on values, attitudes and upbringing that changed over generations. Age group 1 (17-34 years) consisted of 31 (15.5 per cent) patients, age group 2 (35-50 years) of 49 (24.5 per cent) patients, age group 3 (51-65 years) of 64 (32.0 per cent) patients and age group 4 (66-87) of 56 (28.0 per cent) patients. The range of stay in hospital was between 3 and 150 days, most of the patients were interviewed on their third day (39 patients, 19.5 per cent), their fourth day (21 patients, 10.5 per cent) and on their fifth day (22 patients, 11.0 per cent). Most of the patients (114; 57.0 per cent) stayed in two-bed-rooms, 46 (23.0 per cent) in four-bed-rooms, 25 (12.5 per cent) in a 3-bed-room, 13 (6.5 per cent) occupied a single room and 2 (1.0 per cent) stayed in a 4-bed-room with an additional fifth bed. 112 (56.0 per cent) were surgical patients, 58 (29.0 per cent) medical patients, 30 (15.0 per cent) were on the oncological ward. This difference occurred because the stay on the surgical wards was much shorter.

Whenever the researcher went there, there were some new patients, in contrast to the medical ward. Due to repeated short-term treatments on the oncological ward, some patients who had participated in the study were readmitted and had to be excluded from the sample. Only 77 (38.5 per cent) patients were located in the recently built wing, 123 (61.5 per cent) patients in the older parts of the building.

Results from individual items

Fear of exposure of personal identity

Twelve items of the questionnaire covered the exposure of the patients' personal identity (Table 5.1)

Women found it more embarrassing to be recognized as a hospitalized patient ($p < 0.05$). Also, the older the patients the more they tended to agree with this statement ($r = -0.201$; $p < 0.01$). Again, more women did not like their identity exposed through names or other data at door or bedside ($p < 0.05$) and stated, therefore, that nobody should know of their stay in hospital ($p < 0.05$). The latter item correlated significantly with increasing age ($r = -0.229$; $p < 0.01$). The older patients were the more they wished they did not have to talk about private matters in front of other patients ($r = -0.146$; $p < 0.05$) and the more they stated that personal matters should be discussed in private ($r = -0.171$; $p < 0.05$). A high proportion of women, 74 of a total of 83, found being exposed to strangers or visitors intolerable ($p < 0.001$). The more beds in a room the more interested were the patients in matters concerning their fellow patients ($r = -0.214$; $p < 0.01$).

The younger the patients were the fewer problems they tended to have concerning the privacy with their visitors ($r = -0.229$; $p < 0.01$). Interestingly, the replies to this statement were independent of the number of beds that were in the room. Women tended to be more bothered by fellow patients' visitors than men ($p < 0.05$). The same applied to the increasing age ($r = -0.283$; $p < 0.001$) and, interestingly, to the decreasing number of beds in the room ($r = 0.250$; $p < 0.001$).

Personal autonomy

Five statements based on the interview findings were offered (Table 5.2).

The older the patients were, the more they thought they had to be prepared to be accessible at all times ($r = -0.179$; $p < 0.05$), that patients could never retire ($r = -0.194$; $p < 0.01$), and that privacy in hospital was limited because of institutional regulations ($r = -0.164$; $p < 0.05$). There was a mild positive correlation between the increasing number of beds and disagreement with the latter item ($r = 0.165$; $p < 0.05$). Patients in single rooms felt better informed than those in larger rooms ($r = -0.156$; $p < 0.05$). More patients in the new building agreed with

Table 5.1
'Fear of exposure of personal identity' – patients' views

	SA	A	U	D	SD
It is embarrassing to be recognized as a hospitalized patient	15 7.5%	20 10.0%	2 1.0%	109 54.5%	54 27.0%
It does not matter if data are openly accessible at the bedside or at the door	53 26.5%	73 36.5%	2 1.0%	43 21.5%	29 14.5%
Nobody should know that I am in hospital	57 28.5%	48 24.0%	3 1.5%	54 27.0%	38 19.0%
I often wish that I did not have to talk about private matters in front of other patients	82 41.0%	68 34.0%	2 1.0%	41 20.5%	7 3.5%
I do not mind being exposed to strangers/ visitors in hospital	13 6.5%	34 17.0%	— —	84 42.0%	69 34.5%
I hear their details and they hear mine, it levels out	21 10.5%	75 37.5%	10 5.0%	61 30.5%	33 16.5%
Personal matter should not be discussed in front of others	102 51.0%	71 35.5%	— —	17 8.5%	10 5.0%
I like to know about the other patients in my room	27 13.5%	67 33.5%	13 6.5%	65 32.5%	28 14.0%
It is difficult to have some privacy with visitors	67 33.5%	77 38.5%	4 2.0%	42 21.0%	10 5.0%
Other patients' visitors often get on my nerves	31 15.5%	48 24.0%	8 4.0%	80 40.0%	33 16.5%
A phone call made in the room attracts the attention of all the other patients if they want or not	52 26.0%	84 42.0%	9 4.5%	50 25.0%	5 2.5%
You never know if and how staff talk about you	38 19.0%	87 43.5%	22 11.0%	41 20.5%	12 6.0%

the statement 'as a patient one can never retire' (p<0.01). Interestingly, more people on the old wards stated they would not mind that much the hygienic issues (p<0.01).

Table 5.2
'Personal autonomy' – patients' views

	SA	A	U	D	SD
Patients have to be prepared to be accessible at all times	90 45.0%	76 38.0%	1 0.5%	28 14.0%	5 2.5%
As a patient you can never retire	69 34.5%	69 34.5%	5 2.5%	48 24.0%	9 4.5%
Privacy in hospital is limited because one has to fit into a system and obey its rules	75 37.5%	84 42.0%	—	34 17.0%	7 3.5%
I often wish I was better informed in hospital	57 28.5%	81 40.5%	—	57 28.5%	5 2.5%
Hygienic aspects regarding the utilization of commonly used facilities are of no concern to me	36 18.0%	77 38.5%	1 0.5%	47 23.5%	39 19.5%

Fear of physical exposure
As this aspect was the most widely discussed in the interviews, 20 statements were prepared to elicit the patients' responses (Table 5.3)

The use of common toilets was of more concern to women than men (p<0.01). The younger the patients were the fewer problems they had using a common toilet (r=0.176; p<0.05). However, patients on the oncological ward had the most problems, surgical patients the least (p<0.01). Patients in the new building found the idea of using common toilets very unpleasant (p<0.001). Patients who stayed longest in hospital (mean 16.18 days) had rather more problems (r=0.157; p<0.05). A majority of patients stated that they had no control over other people using the toilet. Patients on the oncological ward agreed most often compared to other wards (p<0.05). Also, more women than men agreed with the statement (p<0.05) and the older the patients were the more likely they agreed (r=-0.155; p<0.05). Patients in the new building agreed more often than those in the old wing (p<0.001).

Table 5.3
'Fear of physical exposure' – patients' views

	SA	A	U	D	SD
I don't mind sharing toilets with other patients	30 15.0%	70 35.0%	2 1.0%	53 26.5%	45 22.5%
One has no control over other people using the toilet	87 43.5%	56 28.0%	7 3.5%	36 18.0%	14 7.0%
A wash-basin in the room is perfectly sufficient	14 7.0%	37 18.5%	1 3.5%	46 23.0%	102 51.0%
I would always try to get a room with en suite facilities	139 69.5%	46 23.0%	2 1.0%	11 5.5%	2 1.0%
It is unpleasant to be washed	63 31.5%	53 26.5%	3 1.5%	62 31.0%	19 9.5%
The worst that could happen to me would be any treatment of the intimate area by another person	77 38.5%	58 29.0%	2 1.0%	53 26.5%	10 5.0%
I don't mind using bedpan/commode because anybody could be in this situation one day	34 17.0%	67 33.5%	1 0.5%	43 21.5%	55 27.5%
One of the most dreadful things would be to use the commode in front of others	105 52.5%	57 28.5%	3 1.5%	28 14.0%	7 3.5%
I would try anything to avoid using a bedpan/commode	116 58.0%	59 29.5%	—	19 9.5%	6 3.0%
Smell and noise are even more embarrassing than being watched sitting on bedpan/commode	111 55.5%	65 32.5%	4 2.0%	15 7.5%	5 2.5%
I don't mind if the contents of collecting bags are visible to anyone	34 17.0%	67 33.5%	2 1.0%	47 23.5%	50 25.0%
I do not differentiate between male and female nurses in assisting me in personal activities	95 47.5%	68 34.0%	3 1.5%	20 10.0%	14 7.0%

Table 5.3 (continued)

	SA	A	U	D	SD
It is better when personal things are done by a nurse of my own sex	56 28.0%	55 27.5%	3 1.5%	72 36.0%	14 7.0%
I don't mind being washed by a nurse of the opposite sex	37 18.5%	88 44.0%	3 1.5%	42 21.0%	30 15.0%
Screens should be used more often	67 33.5%	56 28.0%	16 8.0%	45 22.5%	16 8.0%
Screens are not necessary as in one room all patients are either male or female	30 15.0%	50 25.0%	7 3.5%	65 32.5%	48 24.0%
You can't be sure that people really don't watch you	63 31.5%	70 35.0%	21 10.5%	34 17.0%	12 6.0%
Screening for examinations is not necessary as we all look the same	46 23.0%	65 32.5%	3 1.5%	48 24.0%	38 19.0%
It is very unpleasant to get undressed in front of strangers	42 21.0%	47 23.5%	1 0.5%	90 45.0%	20 10.0%
I find it annoying to have to be always prepared for the fact that in a hospital doors may open without warning	35 17.5%	54 27.0%	4 2.0%	78 39.0%	29 14.5%

Female patients particularly disagreed that a wash-basin in the room was sufficient, and of all, patients in two-bed-rooms disagreed most ($r=-0.214$; $p<0.01$) as did patients in the old building ($p<0.05$). The need for a room with en suite facilities became stronger with increasing age ($r=-0.266$; $p<0.001$) and decreasing number of beds ($r=0.217$; $p<0.01$). The average stay of the 139 patients who strongly agreed was 13.48 ($r=-0.180$; $p<0.05$) indicating that the longer patients stayed in hospital the more the need became not to share common facilities.

Female patients more than male ($p<0.05$) and older patients more than younger ($r=-0.170$; $p<0.05$) found being washed unpleasant. Treatment of the intimate area was also more uncomfortable for women ($p<0.01$) and older patients ($r=-0.224$; $p<0.05$). Particularly older patients stated that they

Table 5.4
'Territoriality' – patients' views

	SA	A	U	D	SD
I wouldn't want a larger room than a two-bed-room	120 60.0%	45 22.5%	—	25 12.5%	10 5.0%
I hope I won't get an additional bed in my room	104 52.5%	57 28.5%	3 1.5%	27 13.5%	9 4.5%
Nurses should knock before entering the room	51 25.5%	46 23.0%	12 6.0%	65 32.5%	26 13.0%
The more patients in a room the less privacy you have	116 58.0%	67 33.5%	2 1.0%	9 4.5%	6 3.0%
Knocking has no effect when people don't wait for an answer	72 36.0%	78 39.0%	10 5.0%	34 17.0%	6 3.0%
I don't like that my toilet articles are practically accessible to anyone	82 41.0%	64 32.0%	4 2.0%	39 19.5%	11 5.5%
Only when I am very ill might the nurses open my bedside locker or wardrobe without permission	106 53.0%	53 26.5%	3 1.5%	32 16.0%	6 3.0%
I generally don't like anybody sitting on my bed	39 19.5%	41 20.5%	4 2.0%	79 39.5%	37 18.5%
Only my family may sit on my bed	45 22.5%	44 22.0%	1 0.5%	66 33.0%	44 22.0%

would try anything to avoid using a bedpan/commode (r=-0.186; p<0.01) and that they found smell and noises even more embarrassing than being watched sitting on bedpan/commode (r=-0.183; p<0.01). More women than men did not like the contents of collection bags being visible to anybody (p<0.01). Women generally preferred female nurses (p<0.001), particularly for personal procedures (p<0.001) and when they had to be washed (p<0.001).

The older patients were the more they preferred screens (r=-0.140; p<0.05). The fewer beds there were in a room the more patients voted for screens (r=-0.169; p<0.05) regardless of the fact that all patients in a room were either male or female. Women trusted other patients less that men (p<0.05) that they would not watch others. Getting undressed in front of strangers was a bigger problem for women (p<0.05), for older patients (r=-0.270; p<0.001) and for patients in smaller rooms (r=0.183; p<0.01). Having to be always prepared for the fact that hospital doors may open without warning concerned more women than men (p<0.05).

Territoriality

Altogether nine questions on territoriality were posed to the patients (Table 5.4).

Women were not in favour of larger rooms than 2-bed-rooms (p<0.05), additional beds (p<0.05), having their toilet articles displayed (p<0.05) and people sitting on their beds (p<0.05). The fewer beds in the room the more the subjects voted for smaller rooms (r=0.481; p<0.001), the more they disliked an additional bed (r=0.280; p<0.001) and the more they stated that larger rooms meant less privacy (r=0.305; p<0.001). With increasing age, patients disliked additional beds (r=-0.245; p<0.001) and found they had less privacy in larger rooms (r=-0.157; p<0.05). They also did not like the fact that their toilet articles were accessible to anyone (r=-0.201; p<0.01) and they were opposed to people sitting on their beds (r=-0.341; p<0.001).

Personal space

This topic was only covered by two questions as personal space did not seem to play such an important role in the interviews (Table 5.5).

Older patients preferred more space around their beds (r=-0.164; p<0.05) and the beds not too close to prevent the spreading of diseases (r=-0.340; p<0.001). Interestingly, the fewer beds in a room the more the patients preferred more space (r=0.158; p<0.05).

Table 5.5
'Personal space' – patients' views

	SA	A	U	D	SD
I like beds not too close because one never knows what disease others have	64 32.0%	61 30.5%	8 4.0%	50 25.0%	17 8.5%
I need quite a bit of space around my bed	57 28.5%	85 42.5%	6 3.0%	39 19.5%	13 6.5%

Effect of invasion of privacy on individual

Effect of invasion of privacy on individual

Five items were prepared to cover the effect of violation of privacy on the patients (Table 5.6).

Table 5.6

'Effect of invasion of privacy on individual' – patients' views

	SA	A	U	D	SD
It is embarrassing to be dependent on others	84 42.0%	62 31.0%	1 0.5%	45 22.5%	8 4.0%
Patients shouldn't make a big fuss about what is done to them, however embarrassing it might be	38 19.0%	77 38.5%	13 6.5%	48 24.0%	24 12.0%
In hospital one has to yield, however embarrassing it might be	87 43.5%	79 39.5%	2 1.0%	26 13.0%	6 3.0%
The sicker one is the less one cares about privacy	99 49.5%	56 28.0%	3 1.5%	27 13.5%	15 7.5%
Patients are forced to do things they would never do in public	92 46.0%	64 32.0%	7 3.5%	32 16.0%	5 2.5%

The feeling of embarrassment through being dependent on others increased with age (r=-0.261; p<0.001) and increasing length of stay (r=-0.153; p<0.05), and decreased with the increasing number of beds (r=0.146; p<0.05). Patients in larger rooms were more likely to agree that patients should not make a big fuss, however embarrassing situations might be (r=-0.146; p<0.05). The necessity to yield in hospital was very strongly felt by patients in age group 4 (r=-0.279; p<0.001). They also felt more than younger patients that they are forced to do things they would never do in public (r=-0.292; p<0.001).

Individual as part of the community

Four questions were used to elicit responses on this aspect (Table 5.7).

The older the patients the more they believed that if the relationship between patients was good it did not matter so much if one's privacy was invaded (r=-0.146; p<0.05), that one's own privacy comes second because one has to consider other patients (r=-0.171; p<0.05), and that conformity is necessary to

Table 5.7
'The individual as part of the community' – patients' views

	SA	A	U	D	SD
When I provide a good example in protecting my fellow patients' privacy they'll do the same in return	30 15.0%	90 45.0%	8 4.0%	58 29.0%	14 7.0%
If the relationship between patients is good, it doesn't matter so much if one's privacy is invaded	82 41.0%	82 41.0%	4 2.0%	27 13.5%	5 2.5%
Your own privacy comes second because you have to consider other patients	65 32.5%	100 50.0%	5 2.5%	27 13.5%	3 1.5%
In certain things like opening the window, there has to be conformity or trouble might be anticipated	100 50.0%	75 37.5%	—	21 10.5%	4 2.0%

avoid trouble (r=-0.286; p<0.001). The room size also played a part in answering the last item. The fewer beds in the room the more patients tended to agree on the importance of conformity (r=0.161; p<0.05).

Coping mechanisms
This topic was covered by three questions (Table 5.8).

Table 5.8
'Coping mechanisms' – patients' views

	SA	A	U	D	SD
When my privacy is invaded, I don't complain but inside I am angry	53 26.5%	78 39.0%	7 3.5%	51 25.5%	11 5.5%
Complaining doesn't help as nobody pays any attention	29 14.5%	31 15.5%	16 8.0%	102 51.0%	22 11.0%
Patients should complain more when they feel their privacy is invaded	65 32.5%	80 40.0%	14 7.0%	35 17.5%	6 3.0%

Women were rather more cautious than men when it came to complaining about violated privacy ($p<0.001$), older patients had also more inhibitions ($r=-0.161$; $p<0.05$). Women doubted more than men ($p<0.01$) that anybody would pay attention to complaints. Also patients in age group 4 (66-87 years) were more suspicious of any benefits of complaining ($r=-0.263$; $p<0.001$). Women felt the need to complain more than men ($p<0.05$) as well as older patients more than younger ($r=-0.255$; $p<0.001$).

Summary

After a description of the participating patients the results were presented under the same themes as were the interview findings. The frequency count of each item was recorded as well as additional scores or information emerging from the statistical tests. In general, the results tended to support the interview findings. Most of the issues that were seen as a problem by the interviewed patients had similar ratings in the questionnaires. This again supports the theory that invasion of privacy and intrusion of territory are of serious concern to hospitalized patients. The next chapter will introduce the development of the ranking scale used in conjunction with the questionnaire.

6 Method 3 – rank-ordering

In this chapter the development of the ranking list will be described, method-ological problems discussed and the method of analysis explained.

Rank-ordering

There is not much literature on the application of rank-ordering as it was used in this study. Generally it can be said that the method is used to generate comparative judgement (Crano and Brewer, 1986) by letting respondents rank a set of items according to a specified criterion. Ranking is certainly subjective (Fleiss, 1981) but some degree of reliability can be assumed as the subjects express their views about a defined topic. Kerlinger (1986) outlined three analytic advantages of the method:
1 scales of individuals can easily be intercorrelated;
2 scale values of a set of stimuli can be calculated using one of the rank-order methods of scaling, and
3 they partially escape stereotyped responses and the tendency to agree with socially desirable items.

Development of the instrument

Stage 1
Based on the literature and the researcher's experience, ten items assumed to be intrusions of privacy were listed on the last page of the interview guide. The items were randomly arranged in the following list:
• others searching through belongings
• others entering the room without knocking
• having to use bedpan/commode

- others sitting on the bed
- having to undress for examinations/dressings
- having to answer questions in front of other patients
- personal hygiene performed by nurse of opposite sex
- beds are too close
- personal belongings are accessible to anybody
- no privacy with visitors

Pilot study. After completing the two pilot interviews the patients were asked to choose the item which would represent the worst invasion of their privacy and label it with '1'. The second worst got '2', and so on. The patient ordered the items and wrote the scores with a pencil on the form provided.

On reading the list of items patients were reluctant to make a clear rank ordering, and in some cases the typed lines were too small to read. The items were re-written on index cards. This enabled the patients to order them and experiment with alternative orderings until satisfied with the result, which was then transferred to the form; but responses were still equivocal. The writing was large for the benefit of elderly patients or patients with poor eyesight. An effort was made to keep the descriptions short. When further explanation was needed, it was ensured that each patient got the same hints. After a retest, the main study was conducted.

Stage 2
On the last page of the Likert scale questionnaire a ranking list was provided, based on the interview results. Some items of the first list had been removed, others added. The items which were removed were:
1 others searching through belongings; the score in stage 1 was high, but this is a rare occurrence.
2 others sitting on the bed; because too many variables and combinations of variables influenced this item ('it depends who...')

Other items were added when they emerged as important themes in the interviews, irrespective of the number of patients mentioning them. In order to keep the list to a manageable size, the items had to be selected carefully. The new list of items was as follows:
- having to share toilets with other patients
- others enter the room without knocking
- having to use bedpan/commode
- having to undress for investigations/dressings
- having to answer questions in front of other patients
- personal hygiene performed by nurses of opposite sex
- no privacy with visitors
- personal belongings are accessible to anyone
- beds are positioned close
- being recognized as a hospitalized patient

103

- being washed
- treatment involving an intimate area of body

Pilot study. When the questionnaire was collected, the ranking procedure was performed with the patient. This time the items were written on index cards from the outset for all patients. The cards were shuffled well before distribution to prevent patients from picking more intruding events and leaving the 'less important' items together in a block without thinking about each item. Ten patients tested the questionnaire with the ranking list. No modifications were necessary and the main study could proceed.

Analysis

The results of the first set of ranked items were calculated manually, firstly, because of the manageable number of items, and secondly, because it was seen as a good learning exercise. First, the mean rank for each item was determined as the sum of the ranks awarded for it by the n patients, divided by n. The corresponding mean ridit was calculated using the following formula:

$$\frac{\text{mean rank} - 0.5}{k}$$

where k is the number of items studied. Using the mean ridit is a convenient descriptive way of presenting rank sums. The term 'ridit' is derived from 'Relative to an Identified Distribution' (Bross, 1958) and is an estimation of the proportion 'of all individuals with a value on the underlying continuum falling at or below the midpoint of each interval' (Fleiss, 1981:151). As statistical tests, the Kendall's Coefficient of Concordance (Hays, 1973:802) and the Friedman Two-Way ANOVA were manually calculated (Friedman, 1937:679).

The data of the second set were analysed together with the data of the Likert-scale items by using SPSS/PC+ software. The analysis consisted of

- frequency counts with Friedman Two-Way ANOVA and Kendall's Coefficient of Concordance W
- cross tabulation ranks by sex with Mann-Whitney-Test
- cross tabulation ranks by age with Spearman Rank Correlation Coefficient
- selection of cases by sex, by age, by sex and age with Kendall W
- the mean ridits were calculated manually

Summary

In this chapter the development of the ranking tool, the method of its application and the procedure of analysis was described. The next chapter will present the results of the ranking procedure of both stages of data collection.

7 Weight of privacy-invading events

In this chapter the results of the rank-order procedure are presented. The first set of data stems from the ranking list attached to the interview guide, the items were based on the researcher's personal experience and the literature. The data of the second stage derived from the list of items based on the findings of the interviews.

Stage 1

List of codes:

A	=	others searching through belongings
B	=	others entering the room without knocking
C	=	having to use bedpan/commode
D	=	others sitting on the bed
E	=	having to undress for investigations/dressings
F	=	having to answer questions in front of other patients
G	=	personal hygiene performed by nurse of opposite sex
H	=	beds are positioned close
I	=	personal belongings are accessible to anyone
J	=	no privacy with visitors

Rank-order (n = 20)

The 20 interviewed patients ranked the 10 items as summarized by the following mean ridits:

C – 0.16
A – 0.315
H – 0.395
G – 0.52
D – 0.535
F – 0.565
B – 0.57
J – 0.60
I – 0.645
E – 0.695

Kendall's Coefficient of Concordance ($W = 0.293$) showed a weak but significant agreement amongst the patients (Friedman Two-Way ANOVA $p<0.001$). The highest agreement would be $W = 1$, the lowest $W = 0$ (Conover, 1980).

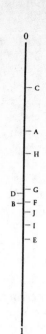

To facilitate an overview of how patients ordered the items, the data may be presented as in Guilford (1954) (Figure 7.1). Figure 7.1 is read as follows: choose an item (for example B) and a rank (for example 3) and read the value where the row and column meet (here 2). This means that two patients ranked the item B (entering the room without knocking) as the third worst (rank 3) of privacy-intruding events.

Rank / Item	1	2	3	4	5	6	7	8	9	10	
A	5	4	3	1	2	2	0	2	1	0	20
B	1	1	2	3	2	2	2	0	3	4	20
C	10	5	2	1	1	0	1	0	0	0	20
D	0	6	1	2	1	1	0	3	1	5	20
E	0	0	2	2	0	0	4	5	3	4	20
F	0	0	3	3	2	2	2	6	2	0	20
G	3	2	1	1	2	3	1	1	3	3	20
H	1	1	5	4	4	3	0	1	1	0	20
I	0	1	1	1	1	3	5	1	6	1	20
J	0	0	0	2	5	4	5	1	0	3	20
	20	20	20	20	20	20	20	20	20	20	

Figure 7.1   Ranking pattern of the 20 interviewed patients

106

Stage 2

List of codes (different from those in stage 1):

A	=	having to share toilets with other patients (*)
B	=	others entering the room without knocking
C	=	having to use bedpan/commode
D	=	having to undress for investigations/dressings
E	=	having to answer questions in front of other patients
F	=	personal hygiene performed by nurse of opposite sex
G	=	no privacy with visitors
H	=	personal belongings are accessible to anyone
I	=	beds are positioned close
J	=	being recognized as a hospitalized patient (*)
K	=	being washed (*)
L	=	treatment involving an intimate area of body (*)
(*)	=	additional items

Rank-order (n = 200)

The 200 patients who participated in the survey ranked the items as summarized by the following mean ridits:

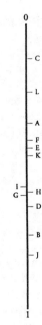

C	–	0.1233
L	–	0.2425
A	–	0.3525
F	–	0.4116
E	–	0.4383
K	–	0.4658
I	–	0.5741
H	–	0.5925
G	–	0.6033
D	–	0.6425
B	–	0.7416
J	–	0.8108

The degree of concordance between patients' rankings was moderate (W = 0.4457), but astronomically significantly different to 0 ($p < 10^{-132}$) because the number of subjects studied is far more than adequate to demonstrate there is some degree of agreement.

107

The following figure represents the patients' ranking pattern, in the same way as in Figure 7.1:

Rank / Item	1	2	3	4	5	6	7	8	9	10	11	12	
A	30	17	38	20	24	20	17	9	7	8	6	4	200
B	2	6	2	8	6	8	13	8	26	25	40	56	200
C	116	45	12	12	4	3	3	2	0	2	1	0	200
D	0	3	5	14	18	16	23	19	23	27	35	17	200
E	5	11	26	23	29	36	23	15	16	8	7	1	200
F	11	10	29	35	24	27	18	18	13	8	3	4	200
G	0	9	5	6	18	22	21	36	29	28	19	7	200
H	7	5	7	13	13	18	23	29	26	30	16	13	200
I	8	9	7	18	14	11	25	27	25	18	28	10	200
J	1	0	5	2	3	6	6	12	17	30	37	81	200
K	2	10	23	29	30	24	23	20	13	13	7	6	200
L	18	75	41	20	17	9	5	5	5	3	1	1	200
	200	200	200	200	200	200	200	200	200	200	200	200	

Figure 7.2   Ranking pattern of the 200 patients

It was decided to examine the patients' ranking according to their sex and age. For more details about the comparison of the rank order by sex, by age, and by sex and age, the author should be contacted. In the following description of the results, the emphasis will be mainly on the first six items in the ranked order because the first items picked were due to the nature of the design the most intrusive events whereas the last items often seemed to be ordered for completeness' sake, and are of less interest. In each case the degree of concordance still differs highly significantly from 0 ($p < 0.001$).

Comparison of patients' ranking by sex

Concordance was rather poorer for male patients ($W = 0.3937$) than for females ($W = 0.5499$), and there was a distinct difference between the rankings. The distance between the items C (having to use bedpan/commode) and L (treatment involving an intimate area), i.e. the difference between the corresponding mean ridits is much smaller for female patients than for male, implying that treatment in intimate areas concerns women much more (0.1833) than men (0.285). Women also seem to feel more uncomfortable (0.33) than men (0.47) when personal hygiene needs are performed by a nurse of the opposite sex (item F). Interestingly, women seemed not to mind so much answering questions in front of other patients (item E; 0.465) whereas men scored 0.4192. Being washed (item K) bothered women more (0.4308) than men (0.49). Having to share toilets (A) was of less concern to women (0.3583) than men (0.3483) (Figure 7.3).

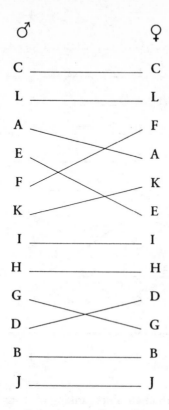

Figure 7.3   Comparison of absolute ranking of items by men and women

Comparison of patients' ranking by age groups

The Kendall Coefficient of Concordance in age group 1 was 0.3937, in age group 2 0.4436, in age group 3 0.4105, and in age group 4 0.5735.

In this comparison it is interesting that the older patients were, the more embarrassing was item C – having to use bedpan/commode – (from age group 1 = 0.1652 to age group 2 = 0.08), the same, although not so obviously, applies to the treatment involving an intimate area – item L – (from age group 1 = 0.2675 to age group 4 = 0.2158). The mean ridit for item K becomes less severe from age group 1 (0.3642) to age group 4 (0.5075) continuously, suggesting that younger people do not like being washed whereas patients in the highest age group do not care so much. Item K occupies the third place in the youngest age group whereas it is in place six in the rest (Figure 7.4).

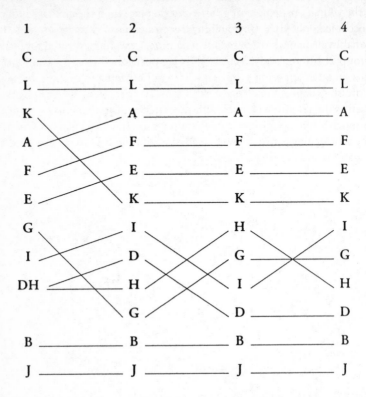

Figure 7.4 Comparison of absolute ranking of items in different age groups

Comparison of male patients' ranking by age groups

While comparing the different age groups one has to consider that the number of cases per group is relatively low. The Kendall W was in age group 1 0.3430, in age group 2 0.3712, in age group 3 0.3666, and in age group 4 0.5536.

Item C was in all age groups rated as the worst privacy-intruding event with age group 3 scoring higher than group 1 and 2, the highest score being in age group 4. Item L shows a slightly increasing tendency, again with the highest scoring in age group 4. Being washed (item K) occupied in age group 1 the third place, the sixth place in age group 2 and 3, the 7.5th in age group 4, indicating that younger male patients would rather not be washed by somebody else. Compared with the other age groups, the younger patients did not mind sharing toilets (item A) as much as did the rest of the subjects, the oldest most. The scores for item E (having to answer questions in front of other patients) went slightly up through the age groups. Having no privacy with their visitors (item G) seemed to concern more the younger patients rating this event on place 6, in the next age groups this item occupied only place 10, 9 and increasing again to 7.5 in age group 4. Item F (personal hygiene performed by a female nurse) was highest rated on place 4 in age group 2. Interestingly, item I (beds are positioned close) was on rank 6 in group 4, in other age groups only rank 8. Item D (having to undress for investigations/dressings) ranked in all age groups rank 10 apart from age group 2 where it was seen as the seventh worst intruding event. The distance between items C and L was much less in age group 2. Age group 4 showed a large gap between item H (personal belongings are accessible to anyone) and item D (having to undress for investigations and dressings) (Figure 7.5).

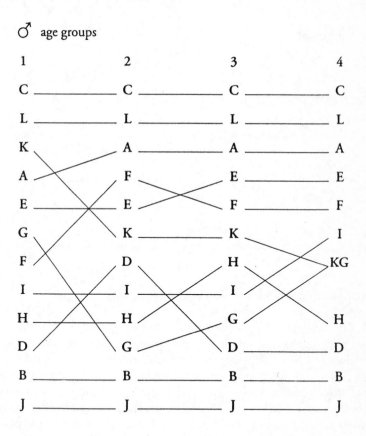

Figure 7.5 Comparison of absolute ranking of items by men in different age groups

Comparison of female patients' ranking by age group

The Kendall W in age group 1 was 0.4771, in age group 2 0.5319, in age group 3 0.5699, and in age group 4 0.6522.

Similar to the male subjects the female patients ranked item C as the worst increasing by the age of the respondents. Again similarly to the men, age group 1 ranked item K third. Item A (sharing toilets) came on rank 3 in age group 2, rank 4 in the others. Personal hygiene performed by a male nurse (item F) was ranked 5 in age group 1, 4 in age group 2, but represented the third worst event in the two last age groups. Having to undress for investigations/dressings (item D) scored its highest rank 6 in age group 1. In this comparison, item B (others entering the room without knocking) ranked last in age group 2 whereas it was usually ranked last on place 11 (Figure 7.6).

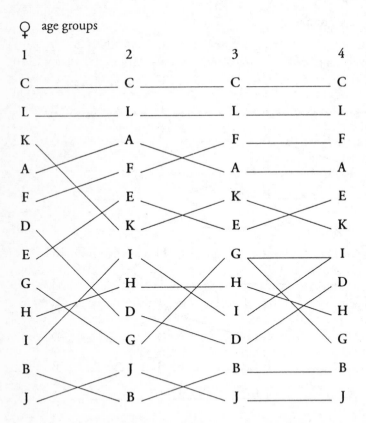

Figure 7.6 Comparison of absolute ranking of items by women in different age groups

General description of the results

Apart from C being the most severe problem in both stages of the ranking, the results of stage one and two cannot be compared meaningfully as a different set of items was used. Therefore, only the second set of results is described here.

Comparing the absolute rank order of all tests, the first two items (C and L) and the last two items (B and J) are generally in a stable position. One has to bear in mind that rank 11 or 12 does not necessarily mean this item does not violate privacy, it just means it is judged the least serious of all offered possibilities. Interestingly, it appears in these comparisons as if a line could be drawn to separate rank 1 to 6 and 7 to 12 into two distinct groups of privacy-intruding events (the first worse than the second): in sex and age-within-sex comparisons, in Figures 7.3 to 7.6, few of the lines joining ranks for the same item cross the horizontal midline.

Another finding is that women seem to have chosen a much closer distance between item C and item L implying that treatment involving intimate areas is for them almost as intolerable as the use of commode or bedpan.

The Kendall's Coefficient of Concordance was highest (>0.53) among female patients. Nevertheless, using the present data and considering the sample size no generalizations can be made to whether male or female patients or patients of certain age groups rank privacy-invading events in a certain manner. However, the resulting patterns can give some hints of different patients' perceptions of privacy in an acute care hospital. A duplication of the procedure with a much larger and more representative sample might prove useful to get more insight regarding interactions with sex and age.

Summary

The purpose of this chapter was to present the data of the rank-order test of both stages of the data collection. An attempt was made to achieve this aim by employing an easily readable way of representing a large amount of data. The findings suggest that all groups of patients rated the use of bedpan/commode and the treatment of intimate areas as the worst privacy-intruding events, while other events such as entering the room without knocking and being recognized as a hospitalized patient, were judged relatively tolerable.

8 A theory of patients' privacy in hospitals

Glaser and Strauss's (1967) distinction between (1) substantive theory which is developed for a specific area, and (2) formal theory which is abstract and is developed on the basis of a substantive theory was seen as very useful to discuss the findings of this study and to attempt to develop their meaning into a general theory. This chapter is dealing with a theory of privacy in hospitals. In Chapter 9 an attempt is made to take this theory onto a more abstract level.

The previous chapters explained the methodology for each stage of the data collection and presented the respective results, structured according to themes which emerged from the interviews. Roughly the same structure will be used in this following chapter, to facilitate an easier understanding of the interpretation of the findings. Triangulation of methods was used in this study to increase its comprehensiveness and to strengthen the results. There were, however, some findings yielded by the different approaches which seemed to be dissimilar or incompatible, and could not be combined simply, a problem acknowledged by Fielding and Fielding (1986). An attempt was made to provide a combined explanation of those controversial findings as suggested by Chesla (1992).

Privacy in hospitals in contrast to home

As could be expected from the lack of definition of privacy in the reviewed literature, the patients were not sure what was meant by this term. Only one patient had protection from body exposure in mind, two thought of data protection, seven, however, linked it with autonomy. Might it be that the lack of autonomy in hospital was so outstanding that it triggered this response? The patients tended to be quite puzzled at the beginning of the interview and they seemed to be rather unfamiliar with the topic. It would appear that no one had ever asked them about this issue. The need for a consideration of this topic became clear, when the patients were questioned about more specific details in the course of the interviews.

That privacy in hospitals is different from home seems to be commonly accepted and the lower the expectation one had the better – results similar to those found by Cartwright (1964), Allekian (1973) and Johnson (1979). Helpless resignation seems to be the response behind these accounts. Be it through previous experience or through hearsay, a stay in hospital has obviously so little attraction that 'one would rather stay at home and suffer more'. It would be interesting to learn what makes children unhappy about the prospect of going into hospital. How do they become 'indoctrinated', and by whom, when such a situation arises? The analogy with a prison illustrates in fact what patients could not express at the beginning of the interview: accessibility of the individual and his belongings, exposure of identity and body, and limited autonomy were the issues determined by established rules in an institutionalized setting.

Fear of exposure of personal identity

Exposure to full view of strangers and probability of recognition
To be recognized as a hospitalized patient could be equated with being recognized as somebody with a fault or imperfection. Ill people usually do not match the image of the young, healthy, successful individual whom we are meant to emulate. More women stated that they wanted their hospital stay to remain secret. When recognized by people of one's own community, the problem seems to be based in the fear of gossip which is beyond the patient's control. A practical example for this is Goffman's (1961) observation that a patient might withdraw when 'he suddenly sees he is about to cross the path of a civilian he happens to know from home' (p.137). The findings of the second stage of this study seem to contradict this assumption. However, this issue was addressed in the very first item of the questionnaire. One cannot be sure how much confidence can be put into those answers, bearing in mind the 'everything is fine' mentality that patients very often display. Having no control over exposure to strangers was seen as a very serious problem. There are numerous occasions in a hospital when patients have to come into contact with 'non-patients'. The entrance hall of a hospital provides an example of this. It still seems to be part of the outside world where 'normal' people have a right to be and can walk around. Patients in their pyjamas and gowns are rather alien elements who due to their role belong on the wards. Belonging to the deviant group of imperfect beings is obviously not a condition one wants to be seen in.

Patients' data at bed or door
Most interviewed patients saw concealed names as a way of protecting their privacy. Again, the threat of gossip and curiosity could thus be minimized. In

stage two, more patients (and more men) stated they would not mind their names being disclosed. Being the second item on the questionnaire, however, it cannot be ruled out that the answer is distorted. That student nurses cannot be trusted was an interesting statement. This finding will be discussed later in this chapter.

Discussion of private matters in front of others
There are many occasions in a hospital when patients have to have a conversation about their own care and other people might overhear this, the ward round certainly being one of the most common events. Patients adopt four different approaches to this issue. The first group of a few patients suggested that they did not mind. The second group of patients thought it did 'not really' matter (meaning it did) because although one has to produce evidence in front of others, the others have to endure the same process, and nobody gets a better deal. The third group thought that at least more private matters should be discussed with the patient concerned alone, the rest of the interviewed patients felt that nothing should ever be discussed in front of others. The distribution of those four categories was indicated by the answers in the second stage, where 75 per cent of the patients wished they could talk in private (but cannot) and almost 90 per cent stated that personal matters should never be discussed in front of others. Being questioned was ranked as the fifth worst intrusion into one's privacy. One important aspect has to be considered here – there is a high probability that a number of patients have questions about their condition but dare not ask in front of others and may go through periods of unnecessary anxiety. For many patients, however, the ward round is the only time they see a doctor. Another embarrassment every patient has to endure is the daily publicly posed question about his bowel activity. Roper, Logan and Tierney (1990) observed:

> ...previously in the patient's adult life no-one has asked daily whether or not he has had a bowel movement. This is a routine in many hospitals and some patients who have not been admitted because of a bowel complaint may well consider this as an invasion of their privacy (p.182).

On the receiving end of the unwarranted conversation were all those patients who said they would not listen (yet – 'one can't help but overhear') or found it embarrassing to listen. In a different context, Goffman (1959) indicated that 'backstage behaviour' is sometimes difficult to maintain due to architectural difficulties (in his example thin walls). He stated further:

> ...here neighbours who may know each other very little find themselves in the embarrassing position of knowing that each knows about the other too well (p.122).

It seemed that individuals who were sensitive themselves thought it must be embarrassing for the patients concerned, and found themselves in an awkward position. An interesting aspect was that – putting privacy aside – some people thought it better to know each other's condition, to share, to help and to comfort others. Patients in larger rooms indicated that they would like to know more details about the others. The reason for this finding might be that patients in a two-bed room usually tell each other on a voluntary basis anyway. A very interesting and certainly underestimated aspect emerged in the claim that individuals participating in the ward round but unknown to the patient create an uncomfortable feeling. Although most probably a member of some authorized group eligible to enter patients' rooms, the anonymity puts him/her on a level with any stranger who must not witness personal matters.

Privacy with visitors
Three quarters of the patients found that they did not have enough privacy with their visitors, particularly acoustic privacy. Even if they said it would not matter, they employed a number of methods to secure at least some form of acoustic isolation. Visitors are a link to the outside world, bringing news, making time pass more quickly. Assuming that patients look forward to at least some of their visitors, even if they do not exchange state secrets they want to talk about all sorts of things no one else needs to know. Those who can get up can leave the room and try to find a quiet place to chat. Bedbound patients are not so fortunate and have to put up with the situation unless their room-mate is kind enough and also mobile enough to leave the room. The size of the room patients were in did not affect their complaints about the lack of privacy, which indicates that it does not make much difference if one pair or four pairs of ears are listening.

Other patients' visitors could be a nuisance, particularly when they were noisy and numerous, and when one sought a little peace and quiet. Interestingly, this applied more to patients in smaller rooms. It seems that visitors' curiosity and activity was easier to tolerate when spread among three or four patients rather than concentrated in a two-bed room. Even if visitors try to whisper in an attempt not to disturb the second patient, this patient might feel awkward being the cause of the inconvenience (having to whisper) but the murmuring itself might be of the same annoyance as normal conversation which is at least understandable. Another reason for this result could be that people who get annoyed by a large number of unknown visitors choose a smaller room as a direct result.

No privacy at the phone
Using a phone in a patients' room posed a serious problem to those sensitive in this area. In order to enable the person on the phone to follow the conversation, it has to be reasonably quiet in the room. This in return

means that it is even easier for the room-mates to overhear at least one side of the conversation, easily making up the other side. How controlled such a conversation must be, knowing that each single word might be scrutinized by an involuntary audience. Faces full of expectation might then force the patient to produce some explanation about the caller and the purpose of the call. With justification one could say, at least the patients *have* a telephone in their room. However, patient care involves more than just the provision of necessities.

Discretion

Patients are undoubtedly at the receiving end in a hospital hierarchy. They have to surrender to so-called experts in the hope that they do know best and will act in the patient's best interest. There may be no sign to indicate how important the patient as an individual is for the staff, but for himself his own interests are certainly primary, particularly in this state of illness. Listening to what Minckley (1968) called 'lighthearted comments' about events regarding other patients most certainly undermines any trust in the staff a patient may have developed. More than 60 per cent of the patients were not sure whether staff might talk about them and what they might say. Laughing and giggling about patients degrades persons to comic objects. Any thoughtless reference to people as work objects could indicate that the person behind the physical entity is forgotten. How damaging it must be to witness such a conversation, not knowing whether one is oneself also an object of mirth.

Personal autonomy

This category was not part of the interview guide but emerged from patients' evidence which indicates its importance to the respondents. An individual's autonomy allows him to act independently and unrestrictedly. Its maintenance seems to be important for a person's psychological well-being. But even if patients' ability to maintain autonomy is reduced by illness, it does not mean that they cannot make decisions about themselves.

Patients play expected roles

People who are admitted to hospital very soon play the role of a patient as expected. Unless they have prior knowledge of how they should behave they learn it very quickly either from fellow patients or from staff. In this way the smooth running of the institution is assured (Freidson, 1970). A majority of interviewed patients felt that privacy in hospital is limited because they have to fit into the system and obey rules. Playing the role of a patient includes the fact that decision making is transferred to the staff and one's own interests seem to have to come last. More than 80 per cent of the patients felt they had to be accessible at all times, almost 70 per cent claimed that they could never withdraw. The patient's own routine has to change, as adaptation is desired. Lack of respect as discussed by Williamson (1992) was also raised. Patients who are not addressed by their own names but by patronizing substitutes feel degraded, depersonalized and not taken seriously. 'One of the most painful experiences of the sickbed is to discover again and again that one has become an object' (van den Berg, 1972b:97).

Lack of choice
Autonomy expresses itself in having choices. Here only the choice of food shall be mentioned since this aspect emerged in the interviews. The palatability of food is an important issue for everybody, all the more so for ill people. Tastes vary and most people prefer food according to their own taste and custom. There are still hospitals which offer no choice of different meals or other variations. Food has to be accepted as it comes from a kitchen designed to suit several hundred individuals. This is reminiscent of the days when coffee was already mixed with milk and sugar in a large jug before being poured into the patients' cups, or bread came with a layer of butter and jam already applied to speed up the process of serving meals times.

Lack of information
A very important aspect which patients linked with autonomy was the provision of adequate information to enable them to make informed decisions. Almost 70 per cent of the patients wished they were better informed. Interestingly, patients in smaller rooms felt better informed. This may be because many patients in single or two-bed rooms are private patients who due to their status trigger a different communication approach. Another explanation could be that patients in smaller rooms have a smaller audience and, therefore, feel more comfortable to ask more – and also more personal – questions.

Lack of control
Lack of control emerged specifically in connection with hygiene. Although half of the patients stated that it was of no concern to them, the other half was aware of the problem with cleanliness and hygiene that occur when so many different people have to share facilities. The fact that these people are ill, incapacitated, unable to care for their personal hygiene as usual, they may even have infectious diseases, aggravates the problem. A perfectly clean environment seems not to be of much comfort when suspicion and distaste make the hospital stay a misery for sensitive people.

Fear of physical exposure

In this study part of the definition of privacy was the determination of private information that is shared with others. Being in full view of others means they get some 'visual' information. A patient who is exposed to other people's gaze has no control over his visual accessibility and experiences shame and embarrassment. Due to its nature, medical and nursing activity requires frequent physical contact with a patient's body with all its imperfections and malfunctions. Activities usually performed behind doors and without spectators – ranging from changing clothes to elimination – suddenly become public issue. As could be expected, this theme was discussed at length and represented the largest part of the findings.

Sanitary facilities in hospital

Older hospital wards usually have rooms with a wash-basin. Three quarter of the patients felt that this was not sufficient for the maintenance of daily hygiene, half of all patients strongly supported this view. Women were in a higher proportion. That patients in the old building shared this view equally could be expected. Patients in two-bed rooms indicated again why they felt so lucky. One problem with the wash-basin was again the hygienic aspect. But there is usually the screening problem as well. Curtains – if available at all – do not close properly, are too short or embrace a much too narrow space which impedes free movement or does not leave enough room for a wheelchair.

Apart from the patients in a single room in the new wing who had their own toilet, all the others had to share either en suite toilets or – in the old part of the hospital – toilets on the corridor. Half of the patients who completed the questionnaire stated that they did not have any problems with that. However, the interviews provided different results in that sharing toilets was seen as awkward, mainly based on suspicion as to the adequacy of the hygiene, and embarrassing. Women did not like sharing toilets with men. In the overall ranking this item was found to be third worst eyent. Interestingly, although women tended to be more sensitive in this matter when filling in the questionnaire, in the ranking this item fell to fourth place, overtaken by 'personal hygiene performed by nurse of opposite sex'. More than 70 per cent found there was no control over who uses the toilets, again, more women shared this view. Patients in the new building agreed more often. One might wonder why, as most of them were accommodated in a two-bed room. These findings have to be seen in the light of the fact that one of the reasons why they wanted a two-bed room was that they did not have to share the toilets with unknown individuals. One patient avoided the dilemma by using the visitors' toilet. Although one might expect the opposite, they were rarely used but cleaned as often as the others and gave, therefore, a fresh and clean impression.

Supporting the above mentioned findings, more than 90 per cent of the patients would always try to get a room with en suite facilities. Patients who had experienced such an arrangement already most firmly wanted the same facilities again. The findings seem also to indicate that patients who stayed longer desired these facilities more urgently. It seems that one can bear shared facilities only for so long. Apart from the fact that only a limited number of known individuals shared en suite facilities, they also represented some environmental improvements for people who could not walk far or who needed more space to enter the bathroom with a walking frame or wheel chair. Unfortunately, through a technical fault the en suite bathrooms in the research hospital were not soundproof and lacked sufficient ventilation. This leads to another aspect. Smell and noise were perceived as very embarrassing, rather a point against en suite toilets. In a shared toilet on the corridor, the user has a fair chance of remaining anonymous whereas in a two-bed room everyone knows who was the cause of embarrassment. This knowledge seems to make the whole affair even worse, a point acknowledged again by the patient who preferred the visitors' toilet. It seems, in his particular situation he got the, for him, best deal. However, despite these technical problems which are the exception, the patients most definitely preferred en suite facilities.

Being washed

More interviewed patients than those whose views were sought by questionnaire stated that they disliked being washed by someone else. It was a more significant problem for women as well as for older patients. Men ranked it as the sixth worst, women as the fifth worst event they could face in hospital. It cannot be concluded from these findings if the problem is the dependence on others performing something one should do by oneself, or if it is related to being touched by strangers or to exposure of the body, the latter point supported by the patient who left 'tricky parts' to be washed by family members. This area certainly needs to be researched more carefully. The degree of the impact of being washed by somebody else on patients was revealed by the evidence of one patient whose temporary indifference towards this event was due solely to his being heavily sedated.

Treatment of intimate areas

The human body seems to consist of two different kinds of parts, some are culturally presentable, others not. Whereas we generally are brought up to cover areas which are called private, in hospital strangers suddenly can claim, and are usually not denied, access to them. Nursing, due to its nature, involves handling parts of the body which are usually only touched in sexual contexts (Lawler, 1991). Be it bathing, investigations or local treatment, several such activities can cause many people considerable stress. It seems the prospect of the procedure itself (such as catheterization) is less threatening than the consequent

121

exposure of the body. This item was ranked second throughout all groups and subgroups. Tasks that are routine for the staff can become a nightmare for the patient to whom this might happen for the first time or at least to which he is not accustomed. Women found it worse than men, older patients generally worse than younger. One way of coping with this situation is the rationale that it is necessary for one's own good or that otherwise a dangerous disease might go undetected. However, these attempts are probably halfhearted and do not really make things easier. Even the 'getting used to it' approach is not very helpful. Getting used to something dreadful does not make it less dreadful in essence. Treatment of this kind will always be necessary. A helpful suggestion for practice might be to limit the number of staff involved in such action and particularly that of students or others who simply want to observe.

Elimination
A function usually performed in private, in hospital elimination can become an event that attracts the concern of other people as well. There is no other socially acceptable area where others are allowed to participate in a person's elimination. From being used to independence, a patient may be forced to use a bedpan or commode, he might need help, elimination becomes a topic for discussion. Being forced to use a bedpan or commode was ranked as by far the worst event that could happen in hospital. The findings of the questionnaire are at first sight puzzling. Half of the patients did not mind the use of bedpan/commode because it could happen to anyone. In the next question, however, 81 per cent stated the use of the commode in front of others would be the most dreadful thing. Following that, almost 90 per cent of the patients agreed (and almost 60 per cent strongly) that they would try anything to avoid using bedpan/commode. It can be assumed that the first question elicited the above mentioned 'it doesn't really matter' – response, whereas the second and third items bring the respondents specifically to the point, the outlined situations seem to be so embarrassing that the respondents felt unable to pass this off as unimportant. The rich findings of the interviews seem to shed light on how patients felt about this topic.

In most cultures elimination is a very personal body function that has to be performed alone in private and out of sight of others. It is an activity inconsistent with our standards of cleanliness, and not a topic for casual communicative encounters. If the fact of its existence were not known, it would hardly be noticeable at all. Patients who need to use a bedpan or commode are no longer able to conform with the social rules. Elimination becomes a highly embarrassing and degrading event. One of the two major problems was the lack of a screen. Being brought up with lockable toilet doors, the visibility or even the slightest possibility of being watched was perceived as almost unbearable. However, even worse was a possible smell. It is not quite clear, whether the only reason for this reaction is the patients' assumption that others might be

122

disturbed by this. The more important reason may well be that the patient might be perceived as somebody whose physical incapacity prevents him from appropriately conforming to accepted rules. Apart from that, the patient is put in a helpless and vulnerable position in which he unintentionally reveals something that is usually concealed. The fact that everybody might be in the same position of vulnerability was not particularly helpful in coping with one's immediate problems. It seemed easier to tolerate when someone else was in this situation rather than oneself. Visitors posed a special problem because they did not belong to the circle of 'insiders' (staff, patients) who had the right to deal with this aspect. Interesting was the answer 'I am not a prude but…'. Whatever the patients' definition of 'prude' may have been, what they meant was in fact that they did mind very much. Using a bedpan was so excruciating for one patient that it even did not matter anymore if a female or a male nurse attended him, an issue that would concern many patients. The degree of embarrassment occasioned by this event is revealed in the finding that although knowing the risk, bedbound patients sometimes try to get up secretly to use the toilet, which is understandable but nevertheless worrying because of its danger. And which nurse has not had the experience of patients limiting food or drink intake in the belief that this will reduce the chance of having to use the bedpan? This practice can be particularly risky for debilitated patients prone to dehydration.

Another aspect of elimination which is often forgotten is the use of collecting bags attached to drains and catheters. There are two possible reasons for embarrassment. One is the fact that urine or other secretions are usually not placed on display. If transparent bags are used, the contents are visible to anyone. Additionally, the actual flow into the bag can be seen. When the bag is opaque with just a transparent section for easier observation by staff, only part of the problem is solved. The second reason for embarrassment might be that the patient cannot control the flow of secretion and is, therefore, seen to be in a helpless position.

Personal tasks performed by nurses of opposite sex
That women felt more inhibited than men when it came to the need to be attended to by a nurse of the opposite sex emerged clearly from the questionnaires as well as from the rank-ordering where men ranked it the fifth, women the third worst event. The first of the three questions regarding this aspect suggested that a vast majority saw no difference between male and female nurses. The findings of the second question differed. It might be that the wording recalled more clearly the patients feelings' and, therefore, triggered a more reliable response. Only one patient commented that this was a control question. Generally, it seems that being washed by a nurse of the opposite sex is not such a big problem for the majority of patients. Male and female nurses have the same training, do the same job, knew in advance what they were undertaking, and are used to it anyway. How far this is used to set the mind at

peace cannot be concluded from these findings. As the ranking suggests, it cannot be that unimportant. Attendance in context with elimination was certainly more distressing than being washed.

There were patients who insisted on being assisted by a nurse of their own sex. An interesting point emerged when two young female patients had contrary views about the relationship between age of female patients and their embarrassment in this context. The findings from the ranking would suggest that the older the patients were the more they preferred female nurses. However, there was a higher proportion of older women in the sample. This question would have to be addressed anew with a stratified sample. It would be interesting to investigate if this aspect can be applied to male doctors as well.

Screens

Lawler (1991) suggested that an important reason for screens was the covering of 'dirty' nursing work. In the German context this seems not to be the case. Screens have disappeared progressively over the last few decades, as was outlined above. Their lack of practicality was said to be one reason for this, there is also the assumption that people are nowadays 'less fussy' than in former times. Questioned about this issue, patients provided a rich variety of data. As could be expected, some people did not mind having no screens. However, as the findings show – more explicitly in the interviews than in the questionnaires – patients were very favourably disposed towards any form of visual barrier which could be used when necessary. Examples were personal hygiene, elimination, having some peace, sleep, avoiding having to see very ill patients. That there were either all men or all women in a room was seen as a rather weak excuse for not using screens. Regarding investigations or dressings, patients displayed a slightly different attitude. Unless the focus of attention was an intimate area, screens were not so crucial as 'we all look the same'. There is, however, one important aspect to consider, which is the uncertainty about fellow patients' attitude and behaviour. There was no guarantee that the others would not watch or at least have a quick look. Women were more suspicious. They seem to be afraid of cruel scrutiny and comparison of their body shapes, an issue that seems not to be so relevant for men. As discussed in previous sections, being watched is everybody's lot and is shared. It seems that accepting visual exposure is in return the price to be paid for watching others, an idea that could be taken so far that patients think they have a right to watch, as one patient stated.

Getting undressed in front of strangers was another embarrassing event. It seems that it is not common practice to leave patients alone when they have to undress. Women again had more problems, probably the same fear of being checked for bodily imperfections as mentioned before, apart from a general reluctance of getting undressed in full view of strangers, even if they belong to the medical or nursing profession. How far the actions of getting undressed and being undressed differ, cannot be concluded from the present findings.

Somewhat surprising at first sight is the finding that patients in smaller rooms tended to demand screens more and also found it more unpleasant to get undressed in front of others. Obviously, the larger the number of potential spectators the worse the situation. As screens were not available, people tried to get a smaller room to at least cut down the number of watchers. In a two-bed room one can negotiate with the second patient or at least have his movements better under control. Summarizing this section, the analysis suggested that screens should be used more often. It also emerged that when the person concerned is passive (such as during investigations/dressings) it did not matter too much being visually exposed. If this body is active (for example when washing or eliminating) it mattered a great deal This can only be a tentative suggestion. The borderline between passive and active would have to be researched thoroughly for clarification of this topic.

Opening doors without warning

This aspect will be discussed again later in the context of territoriality. This section will deal with suddenly opened doors which allow a view of patients who are not in a socially acceptable state, for example, being partly or totally undressed or when using the toilet. Half of the patients did not mind very much; however, this seemed to be applicable only to nurses. Nurses, due to their status, had a right to burst in and see the patient in what he/she would see as embarrassing situations. One obviously has to expect this in hospital. One suggested interpretation of the evidence 'it would be only a nurse anyway' will be presented in a later section of this chapter. There were, however, other patients who were annoyed when nurses saw them in an unpresentable state. Whatever status the nurse may have in the eyes of those patients, the time between the bursting in and the recognition of the intruder may be short but nevertheless enough to cause shock. The consequence is that even for a very short time the patient feels he has no control over his visual accessibility.

Wearing operation gowns

Although operation gowns were practical for some patients and they were usually only worn for a short period, more patients did not feel comfortable knowing that their back was exposed if they did not take precautions. If it was tolerable at all it was in front of fellow patients or staff, but not visitors. Others' sense of privacy was violated when they were forced to see somebody in such a state. A couple chose to discretely look away to spare the blushes of a person in an operation gown.

Active control over one's body

Lack of control over one's body emerged as a source of major concern. In hospital, patients can find themselves in a number of states such as sleep, anaesthesia, coma, in which they do not have any control over how they present

125

themselves to any potential viewer. Goffman (1963) acknowledged the need to maintain a proper composition of the face on waking to be presentable again. This may be applicable to the other above mentioned events as well.

Territoriality

The hospital seems to represent a territory that is rightfully occupied by doctors and nurses. A person's admission to hospital means that – eligible through illness – this person may temporarily claim a small part of somebody else's territory. The respondents had different views about the size of their territory. The range was from 'the bed only' over all possible combinations of bed, bedside table and wardrobe, up to half of the room and equipment in the case of a two-bed room. This reminds us strongly of Altman's (1975) primary territory. In contrast to Altman's theory, patients' primary territories have features of secondary territories as well, namely lack of exclusiveness, and less control. Activities usually performed in primary territory have to be performed in secondary territories. How this affects patients has to be examined more closely. Being a rightful member of the organization 'hospital' (Freidson, 1970), patients occupy places temporarily, such as bathrooms, phone boxes, reading rooms etc. Although public places, the patients seem to have more right to be there than anybody from outside. Their permanent territory is in contrast their bed, bedside table, locker and place for toilet requisites, locations close to oneself and containing personal belongings. The safety of a stable territory allows a feeling of something a 'bit like home'. Territories in hospital also have to be marked. Although hooks are available, dressing gowns are frequently placed across the foot end of the bed. Bedside tables are personalized by photos, flowers and personal belongings. This behaviour is consistent with the social systems regulations, where early marking prevents 'war' (Altman and Chemers, 1980).

Preferred room size
The most desirable arrangement seems to be a two-bed room. A large majority stated they would not want anything larger than that, particularly women. Although the medical profession may not be inclined to agree, private patients go private for the smaller room and enhanced amenities, not for the consultant's treatment. That smaller rooms provide more privacy was emphasised by more than 90 per cent of the respondents. Occupants of small rooms did not want to change to a larger room. There was also much support for single rooms, at least for some peace and quiet. Very ill patients, it was assumed, would, however, be pleased to have a second person in the room for safety reasons.

> [In single rooms] loneliness can become much more frightening than it would be in better circumstances. The mere physical proximity of

other patients with its accompanying sense of shared difficulties serves a useful purpose (Visotsky, Hamburg, Goss and Lebovits, 1961:431).

It is customary in many hospitals to transfer very ill patients to a single room, in the belief that they need their rest but probably meaning that they do not disturb others so much.

Although larger rooms could provide some entertainment – when everyone feels up to it – and companionship, they were less favoured. Men seem not to bother so much, possibly a relict from their military service days.

Structures of dominance in patients' rooms as investigated by Sundstrom and Altman (1974) were recognized in an earlier study by this author (Bauer, 1991). It would be interesting to learn how room size affects the relationship between patients.

Additional bed

Sometimes it is necessary to put an additional bed in a room. Although there was not much one could do about this, a large majority opposed this solution. An additional patient is forced to claim territory that originally belonged to somebody else. The 'first' owner is pushed aside, has to give up part of his space, perhaps even locker space. Probably only the rationale that this was done only in exceptional circumstances prevented patients from employing defence mechanisms. But 'silent' fights can go on with staff unaware of them. Patients in larger rooms did not mind so much. An explanation could be that they had already had to arrange themselves with a number of other people. One more patient probably does not make much difference in this circumstances. Another reason could be that in new two-bed rooms the blueprint is such that everything is designed for two occupants. Sharing two lockers among three patients is not comfortable and may be the source of disharmony. Older larger rooms have no such provisions; although less roomy, it seems much easier to accommodate an additional person.

It comes as no surprise that patients who are forced to join a well established room 'community' do not feel very comfortable about it either. Assuming one's presence to be irritating for others certainly provides the basis for disagreements. Even a pleasant host cannot disguise the fact that one is an intruder. Being at the mercy of others does not help to make things feel any better.

Knocking

It is customary to announce the intrusion of somebody's territory. In the case of entering rooms, people usually knock on the door. It was interesting to learn if the same behaviour is applied to wards, and if so, how this was perceived by the patients. The researcher remembers times when it was not customary to knock at patients' doors, not even those of private patients', as the ward 'belonged' in fact to the nurses. Due to their status and the work that had to be done, they were moving on home territory where it is rather the patients who were the intruders. What we could call common courtesy was not then acknowledged as necessary. Times have changed and door knocking can be observed throughout the hospitals. It seems, however, to depend either on ward policy or on the individual's manners and upbringing.

The patients responded very differently to knocking. About half of the patients preferred knocking, although, as three quarters of all patients negatively commented, it had not much effect because no one waited for an answer. Despite this disadvantage, it was at least a means of warning although not much different from pressing the handle down. Patients tried to explain this habit by the staff's work load and time constraint and also with the inability of some patients to answer. This and the fact that patients feel they don't actually belong here may be the reason for those respondents who did not mind whether nurses knocked or not. The explanation why one patient felt that knocking could even be disturbing, might be because visitors knock the doors and a knock could be associated with a non-staff individual about to enter the room. Therefore, this patient felt frightened unnecessarily. The distinction between patients who perceive the space they occupy as their territory and those who do not, may influence the preference of knocking against the indifference towards it.

Accessibility of belongings

In order to clean a bedside table, the patient's personal items have to be removed. This happens usually while the patient is there and this action did not pose a problem for most of the respondents. When patients remove those items themselves it is usually interpreted as a helpful gesture towards the cleaner. How far it might also be a protection mechanism cannot be concluded from the present findings.

A more serious problem was the fact that toilet articles of every kind were accessible to anyone, either visually or literally. Patients, and particularly women, felt uncomfortable and even disgusted at the thought that someone could use them, either on purpose or inadvertently. A reason for women being so sensitive might be that the viewer could see what potions and devices they used to maintain their appearance, an aspect usually concealed from the public. Although impractical for many reasons, patients preferred to put their mind at rest by storing those items close to them where they could be kept under surveillance. The safety of personal belongings was not a major problem. Patients generally trusted each other and did not lock their wardrobes. A very serious violation of privacy, however, was the opening of bedside table and wardrobe by staff without permission. Only in extreme circumstances, such as inability to give permission, could exceptions be made. As will be recalled, the bedside table and wardrobe were part of a patient's primary territory. The understanding that these places were 'sacred' involved not only fellow patients but also included the staff. It seems easy to forget this when a nurse is involved in her busy routine. How quickly is a locker door opened 'just to get a clean nightie out' not knowing that in this short moment a patient's feeling of privacy was considerably compromised. In this context an interesting issue emerged. Patients pay a small fee for the rent of their telephone. Those phones could also be used by nurses and doctors for internal calls. Although free of charge, taking for granted the use of this facility which a patient considers his own by payment seems to violate his sense of possession. Only one patient raised this issue. It might be anticipated that more patients are confronted with this problem and possibly annoyed.

Occupation of the bed
Another part of a patient's primary territory – and its core – is represented by his bed. Altman and Haythorn (1967) acknowledged the 'inviolability and sanctity of a person's bed, the bedding, and pillow' (p.178). It was for a long time the practice on German hospital wards to sit on the patients' beds, either because this was a more comfortable position to carry out certain nursing tasks or because the intention was to show more sympathy and closeness with the patient during conversation. The relinquishing of this habit was explained by hygienic reasons. Although most of the nurses seem not to sit on beds anymore, doctors can still be found taking uninvited a seat on the patient's bed. The patients' response was equivocal and covered a wide range of combinations of who might – under certain circumstances – and who might not sit down on their bed. Some patients did not like it at all, some allowed family members. Some allowed access to their territory exceptionally if their visitors could not find another place to sit. Hygienic reasons were given as an explanation for exception being taken to this practice; protection of the territory must be assumed. Where the boundaries lie, can only be surmised. The same applies to items that are left on the bed which reminds us of the imaginary patient in van den Berg's (1972b) 'The Psychology of the Sickbed'. Visitors who leave their coats on the bed usually put them exactly where patients mark their beds with their dressing gown. Could this subconsciously be perceived as a take over of one's territory? The same may apply to all sorts of nursing material that is thoughtlessly placed on the bed. Of interest was the idea that if the bed territory had to be intruded upon in this manner (by staff or material), it ought to be for one's own benefit and not for the benefit of another patient in the room. Occupying a patient's bed could be rated not only as an invasion of territory but also as an intrusion into an individual's personal space.

Closeness of people and equipment
A large number of patients seem to prefer quite a large space around their beds, not only because of the uneasy feeling of risk of contagion when in too close proximity to another patient. Older patients needed even more space. Closeness could be perceived as claustrophobic, particularly if it is combined

with feelings of disgust and repulsion towards other patients. Perhaps illness lowers the threshold of tolerance. Closeness that may be acceptable to a healthy person, may be intolerable for an ill person. There has not, however, been any proof up to now for such a proposition. Another interesting aspect was that equipment in use for other patients' and also their visitors are preferably at a greater distance. This suggests that closeness is only accepted when the close individual or object is related to oneself in some way. An idea, we remember in connection with 'sitting on the bed'. Territories are sometimes adjacent to a window or another location frequently used by others such as a wardrobe, table or wash-basin. Depending on a patient's perception of his territory, these numerous intrusions could be experienced as upsetting.

Provided that touch employed by nurses was not 'peculiar' in a sexual sense, the intrusion in what Hall (1966) called intimate space was of no problem to most of the patients. To what extent this reflects having to accept the inevitable, has yet to be investigated in detail. The sample of the patients interviewed was too small to determine similarities to Allekian's (1973) or Lane's (1989) findings of women being less favourably disposed towards touch than men.

Effect of invasion of privacy on individual

Dependence

Dependence on others, staff or patients, poses a major problem to a person who cannot maintain his usual routine or perform usual actions by himself. It was an increasing problem for patients who stayed longer in hospital. Help seems to be easier to accept – although undesirable – only for a short or acute period only. Being a 'nuisance' over a longer period seems to become more awkward. Also patients in smaller rooms felt dependence on others as more uncomfortable. The reason for this could be that pleas for help concentrate on a smaller number of individuals who have – in the end – to help more. Three components of dependence emerged from the data. Patients were concerned about the fact that they were not in control, that they had to bother others, and that help from others focused on embarrassing situations (for example on elimination). Within the variation of each individual case, a combination of all three aspects is highly probable. Here again we find that patients take all sorts of risks in order to avoid dependence. A reason for the dislike of being helped or 'pampered' may be that as a consequence, the individual finds himself automatically in a dependent role.

Patients find themselves in a paradoxical situation. They have to be grateful for something that by its nature is perceived as dreadful. Gratitude towards staff has a high priority. Gratitude that there is somebody who undertakes unpleasant tasks, was often mentioned. However, interestingly enough, it was only mentioned in connection with being washed, never with elimination. Embarrassment in the latter case seems to overpower and paralyse every normal reaction. If one expresses thanks, the focus of the conversation is on something that is not a conventional talking issue. The question of when this transition from being annoyed to being grateful happens, has yet to be researched in detail.

Helplessness
Whatever is done to them and however embarrassing it might be, the vast majority of the respondents saw themselves as totally powerless and without any means of escaping the trap they found themselves in. Older patients felt even more keenly their lack of control. This may be rooted in their traditional upbringing at a time when an individual's assertiveness was not supported. Again a majority felt forced to do degrading things one would never do normally in public, and again more older patients shared this view. In contrast, the opinion that patients should not make such a fuss whatever was done to them, was shared by half of the subjects, more strongly so by those in a larger room. This could be a sign of camaraderie, meaning that all of them are at times in difficult situations, or a warning that it would be a problem if all four or five in one room were fussy.

Helplessness derives from the situation in which extraordinary degree of control is held by one individual over another's physical and social environment (Lazarus, 1966), in this context hospital staff over the patients' environment. Lack of control probably has a negative impact on patients. 'Helplessness adds to the burden of the illness' (Lazarus, 1966:98) and '… further weakens a physically sick person…' (Seligman, 1975:182). Instead of helping a patient, the circumstances compromising his privacy in hospital seem to hinder his recovery or provide additional hardship. As was mentioned elsewhere, a patient is expected to surrender in order to facilitate the smooth running of the institution hospital. The control has to be, therefore, with those who know best, the employed experts. Seligman (1975) called this phenomenon 'institutionalized helplessness' and explained:

> …institutional systems are all too often insensitive to their inhabitants' need for control over important events. The usual doctor-patient relationship is not designed to provide the patient with a sense of control. The doctor knows all, and usually tells little; the patient is expected to sit back 'patiently' and rely on professional help. While such extreme dependency may be helpful to certain patients in some circumstances, a greater degree of control would help others. Being hospitalized, then stripped of control over even simple things – such as when you wake up and what pyjamas to wear, may promote efficiency, but it does not promote health (p.181-2).

The word 'doctor' can easily be substituted by 'nurse'. It is mportant that in almost all statements the term 'control' – or more properly the lack of control – appears. Control means power, the patient has none of it, reflected in Seligman's (1975) theory of helplessness which claims that 'organisms, when exposed to uncontrollable events, learn that responding is futile' (p.74). It is perhaps worthwhile considering for a moment all the bedbound patients who more than anyone else are sentenced to the experience of helplessness. 'The combination of helplessness, lack of technical competence and emotional disturbance make him [the patient] a peculiarly vulnerable object for exploitation' (Parsons, 1951:445). One could thus argue that the degree of nurses' responsibility to protect a patient's privacy grows proportionally with the degree of patients' dependence.

Severe illness leads to capitulation
The threshold of one's need for privacy is set much lower if a severe illness with its consequent inability to maintain an appropriate self-presentation occurs. Extreme physical helplessness seems to influence the psychological feeling of shame or embarrassment. Obviously, three stages emerge. First, a healthy person experiences embarrassment if he does not present himself or conduct himself properly. Second, the same applies to an ill individual who is mentally awake. Third, if a patient is seriously ill, the physical incapacity of his body overpowers his mental control and, therefore, any need of privacy is abolished. There was a small minority of respondents who disagreed with this view. There might be individuals for whom the breach of privacy takes on such dimensions that they would cling to its maintenance with all the strength they have left. Another explanation is that they had never before been very ill, so that they had not had the experience to be able to judge their behaviour under such circumstances.

The individual as part of a patient community

Ingham (1978) suggested that in a good relationship between individuals privacy becomes more flexibly handled over time on a voluntary basis. This idea was supported by a large majority of patients. Harmony between individuals seems to soothe situations that might otherwise be insurmountable. The assumption of many respondents was that 'good' behaviour could be expected and would be granted in return, based on mutual tolerance, understanding and sympathy. Wishful thinking (it cannot be what should not be) may be part of the coping mechanism that allows one to put one's mind at rest by assuming the best. Doubts remain as to how far the widely emphasized consideration for others is genuine or simply 'part of the deal'. In order to maintain a harmonious coexistence, regulations for public behaviour as expressed by Goffman (1963) have to be employed. Conformity among patients had to be achieved to avoid serious trouble. The interesting finding was that people in smaller rooms emphasized conformity more. The explanation might be that patients in a larger room could get away with agreeing or disagreeing with their room mates' opinions or wishes or simply being indifferent if they so wished. In a two-bed room there is only one other 'protagonist' who can by no means remain anonymous but has to express an opinion. Which sanctions are employed for unsuitable behaviour could not be established. However, it seems that the single room could be used as a weapon for people who cannot conform or who behave inappropriately. The inability to pay expensive insurance is used as a means to make others adapt and behave accordingly ('if you can't pay you have to stay with us and shut up'). It would be interesting to learn where the foundations of good relationships between patients are between being genuine or being a necessity. The importance of matching patients in rooms is highlighted by the above mentioned evidence.

Reaction to invasion of privacy and coping mechanisms

Schuster (1976a) developed a model of interpersonal distancing with the behaviour of withdrawal/retreat on one end of the continuum and disclosure/communication on the other, depending on the individual's need in an individual situation. She acknowledged that physical distancing is less easy to maintain in hospitals than in other circumstances, as did Shumaker and Reizenstein (1982): 'coping strategies available to patients who have inadequate control over their privacy within hospitals are severely limited' (p.206). Despite these difficulties, the most popular method to deal with invasions of privacy seems to be retreat. The effort to avoid confrontation with unpleasant situations or persons was represented in actions such as moving to another room, not maintaining contact with potential intruders, trying to find an acceptable solution. Others withdrew by covering themselves or hiding under the blanket in an attempt to isolate themselves from the hostile environment. Certainly one of the most worrying methods is self-discharge against medical advice. If these actions are not successful, the majority of patients surrender angrily, women and older patients more so. This supports Lorber's (1979) findings of older patients being more submissive. Whether this is demonstrated as polite resistance or as aggressive rejection of care depends on the patient's personality. Complaining seems not to be a popular method. A third of the respondents thought it would be useless anyway because nobody would care. Others felt it could be perceived as offensive, although complaining would be the right thing to do, as almost three quarters of the respondents stated. Women and older patients who were more likely to give in angrily, wished they had the courage to complain. Reluctance to complain is similar to French's (1979) findings, where respondents took the onus upon themselves rather than blaming the hospital for lack of privacy. One must assume that in return for all the work nurses do, the least one can do is not to criticize. Nehring and Geach (1973) suggested that this persistent reluctance to complain arose out of fear of reprisal. It seems that 20 years later patients have not become any more assertive and aware of their rights. But then again, how can one complain when one has to be grateful? There seems, however, to be a limit to tolerance. Consideration for others and respect for staff goes only so far. If things get too bad, action has to be taken. In these exceptional circumstances patients risk complaints knowing they might not be seen favourably by the staff. Recalling the literature on 'unpopular' patients (for example Stockwell, 1984), complaining was seen as one of the features of 'bad' patients. When approaching one particular patient for an interview, staff had warned that he would be a 'complainer'. It turned out that he criticized a lot that he found wrong. The researcher was pleased to hear 'true' evidence of a patient's perceptions, staff were not. Under these circumstances it is not surprising that patients keep quiet for the time being, in the hope of pleasing staff in an attempt to make sure of receiving the care staff thinks is suitable, and look forward to the time of discharge when the nightmare comes to an end. This is another consequence of their dependence as discussed earlier. This explains also why many patients did not know what to change although the evidence invited some comment in this direction. If suggestions were made at all, they concerned environmental features, for which no one but an anonymous architect was to blame. Only very few aspects which depended on currently employed and visible people were criticized.

A theoretical concept of patients' privacy in hospital

Parsons' (1951) description of a patient shall introduce this section:

> ... he is cut off from his normal spheres of activity, and many of his normal enjoyments. He is often humiliated by his incapacity to function normally. His social relationships are disrupted to a greater or a less degree. He may have to bear discomfort or pain which is hard to bear, and he may have to face serious alterations of his prospects for the future, in the extreme but by no means uncommon case the termination of his life (p.443).

Who is this unfortunate individual who has to come to hospital and is confronted with so much hardship? Who is this person who has to put up with an often radical change of privacy? Patients bring a whole set of characteristics to the setting: age, sex, circumstances of upbringing, previous hospital experience, hearsay and probably even family size or living conditions, which all seem to be significant in their influence on the need for privacy. A patient's reaction to invasions of his privacy is, however, also affected by those factors. Culture has an important influence over some of those factors and has, therefore, to be cited as well. This does not only apply to foreign patients but, congruent with MacGregor (1976), also to patients who come from different regions within one country, be the difference geographical, ethnic or between urban and rural settings. Different social backgrounds play an important role as well.

A variety of properties of theories of privacy and territoriality discussed in the literature seem to be reflected in the findings of this research project. The theory of personal space – or more precisely intimate space – does not seem to have the importance in hospital that it has in day-to-day encounters. Intrusions due to diagnosis and treatment are anticipated and do not, in general, pose a serious problem. Supporting Allekian's (1973) assumptions, intrusions into personal space in hospital are not as anxiety provoking as might be expected.

Schuster (1976b) identified four factors that play a role in a patient's perception of his privacy:
1 level of consciousness and awareness,
2 specific character of patient-to-patient relationship,
3 mobility (helplessness), and
4 perception of role.
All those aspects are recognizable in the data yielded by this present study. The key factor in the perception of privacy seems, however, to be the degree of control a patient has. Control correlates with power. If control is taken away, for example through institutional regulations, physical or mental incapacity or for other reasons, the patient becomes powerless. The mutual relationship of a positive or negative feeling of control seems to be correlating with the positive or negative perception of integrity of privacy.

To prevent this state of powerlessness, the desired level of privacy has to be maintained. An acceptable degree of control has to be preserved and a wide range of regulation-mechanisms (privacy) and/or defence-mechanisms (territory) have to be employed. It must be assumed that failure to maintain privacy ('one can't help ...') is detrimental to a person's well-being. In the hospital context, it may aggravate psychological or physiological disturbances. This, however, is not what we would wish to happen. Applicable here is Florence Nightingale's axiom that, at the very least, hospitals should not make patients worse.

The model (Figure 8.1) shows an interesting relationship of variables across the categories privacy, territoriality and behaviour. It illustrates the effect of the patient's need for privacy (influenced by a number of factors such as age, sex, upbringing, culture and so on) on the perception of the territory he occupies while hospitalized, and on his subsequent behaviour as well as the staff's assessment of this behaviour.

135

Engagement in regulation- and defence-behaviour is also influenced by the identity of the invading individual. There seem to be different levels of acceptable audience.

Staff, due to their insider-status, are allowed to be very close to the patient and also perform activities which would not be accepted outside the medical context. Trust has an obvious influence on the distinction between permitted staff. A question that has to be answered is, for example, what attributes does a nurse have to have to be seen as trustworthy? Student nurses do not yet quite belong to the established staff and have to be treated with caution by the patient. Until they are formally admitted to the profession, they still belong more to the outside world ('civilians') and are viewed from a different perspective. An interesting thought emerged during the interpretation of the data. Nurses who burst into rooms or bathrooms without knocking might be forgiven for invading privacy. Apart from the question on whose territory they are moving, an explanation could be that patients feel nurses are closer to them than doctors (who knock). The remark 'it would only be a nurse anyway', however, reminds us also of the servants in former times. They were seen as non-persons, who did not solicit the effort of 'front stage behaviour' from their masters. The nurses' reaction to being perceived as a non-person would have to be explored further. Other patients are an acceptable audience in so far as there is a harmonious relationship amongst them, although there are limitations as to what they are allowed to share. As they may see themselves as being in the same boat, their shared struggle to survive in the system makes a lowering of the restrictions that protect their privacy more likely. Visitors belong in fact to the outside world and only their relationship to one of the fellow patients may trigger some allowances, total strangers or passers-by have no right to invade a patient's privacy in any way. Family members seem to have a special status, depending on their relationship with the patient and on their usual closeness and behaviour among themselves at home. As a consequence, sometimes they can be readily accepted where nurses might not be whereas on other occasions they may be sent out of the room like any other stranger when rather 'delicate' procedures have to be performed. The fact that a baby boy was bathed by his mother hundreds of times does not necessarily mean that he enjoys the same action when he is grown up.

In summary, one can assume that there is a distance continuum of acceptable audience from staff to stranger with the family member as a freelance element (Figure 8.2):

There seems to be a clear hierarchy of acceptability of intruders, but the number of those individuals represents a further variable in the decision to grant access. For example, one or two nurses having to intrude upon a patient's privacy are readily accepted because of the above mentioned reasons. Increases in the number of nurses pose a threat which seems to cancel out the privilege normally granted to staff. The level of acquaintance seems also to be a crucial

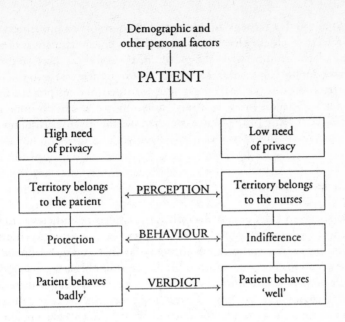

Figure 8.1   Diagram representing the variables involved in patients' privacy-protecting behaviour

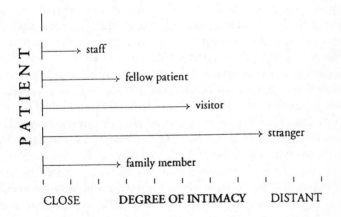

Figure 8.2   Diagrammatic representation of the relative degree of intimacy

point. Some prefer rather anonymous and, therefore, neutral persons for 'difficult' tasks where they feel there is no need for embarrassment as there is no personal relationship between the parties. Others feel the need to develop a certain amount of trust to allow somebody access to their body.

Apart from the distinction of acceptable intruders in one's privacy, a certain mental capacity seems to be necessary to maintain and express one's need of privacy. If the severity of the illness overshadows the psychological aspect, the level of tolerance of invasions raises considerably.

Implications for nursing

In the first stage of the data collection for this project a phenomenological approach was adopted because it seemed to be the most appropriate way of understanding the life-world of the informant as experienced by the individual concerned. After making the effort of understanding this experience, it would seem unreasonable not to use the same approach when dealing with patients in practice. If we put ourselves more often in the patients' shoes, our daily practice would be more influenced by individual understanding and less by textbook-guidelines. This view is taken when the following aspects are discussed.

It seems not to be the case that a society's gradual changes in attitudes and morals automatically include everyone. Screens that disappeared over time may serve as an example. This disappearance obviously did not reflect the actual needs of the patients concerned, who felt very uncomfortable when physically exposed. It seems high time to make their presence on the wards so self-evident that patients who want them do not have to be afraid of being seen as prudish or old fashioned. How far the observed so-called thoughtless intrusions into patients' privacy by professionals are indeed thoughtless has yet to be clarified. The fact that private patients receive a different treatment shows that there is some appreciation of the need for privacy, even if it is expressed in a selective mode. The deliberate invasion of the patient's privacy could be seen as a way of expressing staff power targeted at the defenceless 'normal' patient.

There seems to be a common notion among nurses that women and/or older patients are generally more sensitive with regard to invasions of their privacy. Men are perceived as rather easy-going in this respect. This study indicates that there might be some trends in the perception of privacy depending on age and gender. It would be easy to compile a list of all the variables used in this study with each single result as a guideline. However, a word of caution is necessary. As individual human beings differ, so do the possible combinations of factors that influence their need for privacy, and also expressions of this need. An age or sex label does not tell anyone how this particular patient may feel about his privacy. Thus there might be a danger that younger people, for example, may feel they are expected to behave in a particular way, and consequently do not dare to complain.

Another assumption is that patients from rural areas care less about their privacy because they have had a harsher upbringing; or, on the other hand, that they are more sensitive because traditional, moral and religious values still have more importance to them than to urban citizens. If we have no knowledge about the concept of privacy and the mechanisms of regulation, and if we are not good observers, we cannot necessarily recognize who is embarrassed and who is not.

Based on the knowledge that control is the key factor in the way privacy is perceived, interaction with patients has to start here. In order to give the patient the feeling that his need for control is satisfied, any actions that could invade his privacy should be adequately explained. This information enables the patient to understand the necessity for the invasion and allows him to make the informed decision to allow access to his self/body. Permission granted is, however, not effective indefinitely. Situations change continuously and with this the need for negotiations with the patient is enhanced. If he feels very ill and weak, his privacy threshold might be lower because he is in need of help and he accepts that this help involves invasion of his privacy. When he feels better, his need for privacy approaches the normal degree again and any potentially intrusive nursing action has to be negotiated anew.

This shows clearly that one cannot give guidelines for the interaction with patients that will suit everybody. For each individual patient in any individual situation, access to him has to be discussed and deliberated. The safest method is to treat every patient as if he/she is the most sensitive individual. It is also necessary to assure the patient that it is perfectly acceptable to state his personal preferences without fear of reprisal. The creation and maintenance of a powerless subculture of patients cannot be the aim of modern nursing.

Protection of privacy does not hurt those who do not care but it means the world to those who do.

Summary

This chapter outlined a substantive theory of patients' privacy in hospital, based on the findings of the different stages of this study. Much of the patients' evidence matched the expectations created in the propositions made in general theories on privacy and territoriality.

Important aspects for patients were the exposure of their identity and the often necessary physical exposure, particularly related to personal hygiene and elimination. Lack of personal autonomy, reflected in the lack of information, choice and control, posed another problem. Patients also reported their need for their own territory, even if this was only temporary. Issues of personal space were surprisingly less important. The knowledge that, due to its nature, medical and nursing action had to be performed very close to the body, prevented the creation of wrong expectations.

The role a patient plays as part of the ward-community was discussed as well as the detrimental effect of the intrusion of privacy on the patient which resulted in feelings of dependence, helplessness and capitulation. Patients seem to construct a hierarchy of acceptable distances to potential intruders with staff allowed closest, then fellow patients, visitors and, farthest away, strangers. The special role of family members was outlined. Similar to the known privacy-regulation mechanisms, patients try to employ certain behaviours to maintain the desired level of privacy and to permit or deny access to themselves and/or their bodies.

Finally, the implications of this theory for nursing were discussed stressing the necessity for continuous individual negotiations to maintain on the one hand the patient's need to feel in control and on the other hand to gain permission for access to carry out the necessary nursing actions. This substantive theory represents the germ of a formal theory of privacy which is delineated in the next chapter.

9 Towards a formal theory of the concept of privacy

This chapter offers an attempt to generate a theory of the perception of privacy which is – although substantively based on the hospital context – applicable to other settings as well. One could argue that it is rather early to do so because it would be based mainly on phenomenological data which – by their nature – apply only to the informants concerned. Van Manen (1990) compared phenomenological study to a poem and stated:

> ...as in poetry, it is inappropriate to ask for a conclusion or a summary of a phenomenological study. To summarize a poem in order to present the result would destroy the result because the poem itself is the result (p.13).

However, an attempt is made to indicate in which direction a formal theory might develop. Subsequently, this tentative theoretical structure will have to be tested. Suggestions of several ways to do this are discussed below.

In the following discussion, the term 'privacy' will be used for the complex phenomenon which includes related areas such as territoriality, personal space, crowding and so on, as it would be perceived and represented by each single individual. This decision was made considering Dubin's (1978) classification of concepts, which he named units. In his taxonomy, privacy would represent a summational unit. Its central attribute is that 'it seems to draw together a number of different properties of a thing and gives them a label that highlights one of the more important' (p.66). The determination of such a unit or concept is the first step in formalizing a theory. The second step is to determine propositions which describe or link those concepts (Fawcett and Downs, 1992). This chapter tries to delineate some possible propositions.

A discussion is offered on
1   how privacy as a subjective feeling is related to the self,

2 the aspect of control over exposure (psychological and physical), over territory and space, and over the acceptability of potential intruders, and
3 coping behaviour.

'Self' and privacy

This last chapter is concerned with the privacy of the individual, not with the privacy of groups, although one can assume certain parallels between the two. It is not the intention here to undertake a thorough discussion of the concept of 'self'; rather the aim is to indicate the individuality of the concept of privacy.

Each individual perceives himself as an entity of exclusive uniqueness and importance. This feeling of 'self', however, rarely has a meaning if there are no others from whom we distinguish ourselves. Only the interaction with others, probably based on intellect, creates the self. Since everywhere in the world individuals are in social contact with others, all individuals have a need for privacy. If there were only one single human being in this world, it would be questionable whether he could have a feeling of self. Mead (1934) suggested that

> ...the self is something which has a development; it is not initially there, at birth, but arises in the process of social experience and activity, that is, develops in the given individual as a result of his relations to that process as a whole and to other individuals within that process (p.135).

The very centre of the self – or 'core self' as Goffman (1959) called it – has to be preserved by all means. Invisible psychological boundaries and barriers exclude or permit access at various levels. Aspects of the self to which no other should have access, are called private. The degree to which this perception of privacy goes depends on how strongly the individual feels about his self, and subsequently also on his self-esteem. A number of factors and variables make up a set of characteristics unique to the individual which influences the perception of privacy. Therefore, the perception of privacy is always subjective. Subjective experience is any experience to which we alone have access (Mead, 1934). The feeling of privacy is concentrated only on areas which are important to the individual. However, and here social interaction plays a role, whatever we do to maintain the desired level of privacy, we can only achieve it if others allow us to have it (Brill, 1990). Sensitive human beings, as social creatures, not only have a certain attitude towards their own privacy but also are sensitive towards the privacy of others. Violation of others' privacy is perceived as being as painful as violation of their own.

The existence of the self makes the human being what he is, therefore, it has to be carefully maintained. Depending on the perception of self and of the attached body, the individual is concerned with how the image of the self is presented to others. Permanent social interaction with others poses a constant danger to the integrity of the self. Each encounter has to be assessed individually and depending on the outcome of this assessment, permission for access is granted or denied. However, each individual breaks the concept of privacy up into a variety of aspects, valid only to himself, because what one person perceives as private might not be of the same importance to someone else. For example, one person might be very concerned about the protection of personal data, yet rather careless about the protection of his body and completely unconcerned about invasions of his territory. Another individual's main concern, however, might be protection from physical exposure and from violation of his personal space, but he can easily tolerate the loss of control in other areas. This differentiates the basis for the above mentioned assessment which in turn leads to negotiations of accessibility to the different aspects of self.

Westin's (1967) four functions of privacy: personal autonomy, emotional release, self-evaluation and protected communication, seem to be very important strategies in the maintenance of the self. If the self develops over time as Mead (1934) stated, this is certainly a slow process. Rapid changes cannot be expected. This means subsequently that alterations of the perception of privacy also do not change quickly. A society's standards and morals change over time, and sometimes this can be quite quick, a change in the individual's perception of his privacy does not necessarily follow.

Control

The key factor in the perception of self is control. Control is a sign of autonomy and reflects power. Features of control can be seen as choice, independence, information, freedom from interference and self-determination. In connection with privacy, control means the ability to either permit or deny access to aspects of self. Referring to Chapter 8, the feeling of being in control positively influences the perception of an inviolate privacy whereas loss of control means the necessity of being on the alert for potential invasions of privacy.

Situations can occur in which the individual loses control for a number of reasons. Control is handed over to or taken from other authorities, such as in hospitals, prisons, homes, or under particular political circumstances. Suddenly, the individual can no longer decide who has access to him and to which particular aspect of his self. Loss of control means helplessness and dependence, situations that are not compatible with self-integrity and self-esteem.

This is also the reason why accepting help is so difficult for many people. We generally value independence highly but there are times when restricted independence is for one's own good. If a person who is used to being independent becomes, for example, disabled, rejection of help could prove to be very harmful. Another problem is that we have no control over what other people do with the information they get about us. Apart from the professional context, where we hope that our trust in the professionals is justified and that codes of conduct are followed, we cannot rely on another's discretion and loyalty.

There seems to be a close relationship between control and trust. As soon as the decision is made, based on information and subsequent negotiations, as to how far and under which circumstances access is granted, the party who is the target of the invasion confidently shows trust towards the invading party that negotiated boundaries will not be infringed. Control is handed over to the potential invader but under negotiated presuppositions. In the professional context, we enter this 'contract' by turning to a professional for help. However, we cannot necessarily be sure that other people consider our privacy because we have not negotiated the terms and have, therefore, no control over their actions.

In conclusion, an individual's perception of privacy is closely linked with the perception of the level of control he has. Three main issues where control plays an important part are discussed below.

Exposure

As there are two entirely different types of exposure, exposure of identity and physical exposure, they are discussed separately.

Exposure of identity. As mentioned above, the self consists of different aspects that are protected from access through others. Private thoughts and feelings are not meant to be revealed to individuals other than those who have permission to participate. Restricted and protected communication, be it spoken, written or on audio-visual devices, is one way of narrowing down the number of potential intruders. Transmission of any sort of private data about the individual is in fact not only a revelation of those data but a revelation of the self of which those data are an inseparable part. Likewise, the recognition of oneself by others in various locations unveils certain information about oneself, for example, in the hospital, the red light area of the town or the 'soup kitchen'. Being seen there implies deviance and being in the wrong. No one would mind being seen at a prestigious sporting event or while shopping in the most expensive boutique in town. The transmission of information in these cases can be either valued and encouraged or feared.

Physical exposure. Transmission of data does not only apply to data in the usual sense such as descriptive personal information, but also to visual and/or acoustic information. In most cultures parts of the human body are covered by clothes of fabric or similar material. This is not only a protection against hostile environmental influences but also a protection of certain parts of the body that are surrounded by an aura of inaccessibility and aptly called private. We do not find it seemly to uncover these areas in normal day-to-day encounters.

Part of the self is, to be able to maintain a socially acceptable presentation of the body. This includes being properly dressed, being in control of posture and gesture, and refraining from impolite, deviant or embarrassing behaviour. Visual accessibility while being in an unpresentable state destroys the sense of the inviolate self. Even the slightest possibility of being watched may lead to insecurity and uneasiness. Intimate body areas as such and everything in connection with elimination are the last things we are prepared to expose to others. However, there seems to be a distinction between being seen in a passive role and being seen as an active agent. Visual access during the act of getting undressed, being washed or during elimination is perceived as worse than during the state of being undressed, being treated or examined. How far a sexual component plays a role in the permission or denial of visual access, has yet to be established.

Territory and space
An individual's perception of privacy does not depend only on the integrity of self-related issues but also on the possession of a personal identified territory and on control over it. Demarcation lines are used not only as barriers to the outside world but also as an embracing safety belt for everything within those boundaries. Anyone who desires admission has to employ conventional means such as knocking, ringing the bell, calling the name of the rightful owner and so on. It is then at the owner's discretion to allow access or not. Entering a territory without permission is a serious offence as are any changes in the environment without the owner's permission. Personal belongings are perceived as being safe as long as they are within the marked territory and in their rightful place. There are differences in the degree to which belongings are private, similarly to the aspect of the self they represent and depending on the relationship between the items and the individual. Letters, photographs, diaries that have to do with the most inner areas of the self are not easily accessible whereas other items such as furniture or clothes are expected to come into contact with others and are, therefore, not in such urgent need of protection. It is difficult to obtain one's own territory but it is also stressful being forced to share another's territory.

Intrusions do not only happen into one's marked area but also across one's psychological barriers. If a person comes closer to another than the latter wants, a person's feeling of self-determination and autonomy is disturbed. Physical distancing is important in the maintenance of the psychological 'self'. Evidence from the literature on personal space suggests that touch is perceived as an intrusion into one's intimate zone. From the evidence obtained in this study on patients, however, this proposition cannot be confirmed. The reason for this may lie in the particular circumstances in which patients find themselves, as discussed in the previous chapter. How far touch is generally a problem, would have to be examined further.

145

Levels of audience

Although access to the self has to be carefully supervised, there are differences in the potential intruders. Depending on the relationship between the individual and the other, the approach may be close or has to remain distant. People who may come closer are either those who maintain a good personal relationship with the individual or are rationally accepted due to their professional status. Unknown or disliked persons are excluded from any access. Therefore, intrusion into one's privacy can be granted as a privilege or taken in the form of aggression and violation. If the relationship between two individuals is good, information is voluntarily transmitted and the need for privacy decreases over time. If strangers are forced to share some time together (in hotels, hospitals and so on) there is the unspoken expectation that everybody behaves according to the rules and does not embarrass one another, silently hoping that no confrontation is imminent.

Altman (1975) distinguished between three types of territories, primary, secondary and public, dependent on the degree of intensity of use and also of the control the occupant has over this determined area. But one could argue that this classification not only depends on the actual physical entity but also on the potential intruder. A person's neighbourhood street may generally be his secondary territory but it becomes his primary territory if residents of another neighbourhood street occupy the first. The number of watchers, listeners or intruders plays a part in the decision of granting access or not, but the hierarchy of acceptable audiences according to their relationship with and closeness to the individual seems to be more important.

Coping behaviour

According to Altman (1975) it is not only exclusion or inclusion of others that is necessary to maintain self-esteem but it is also the ability to regulate and to control the desired level of contact. A problem arises when the defence and regulation mechanisms do not work, mainly because control is handed over to someone else or taken by them. Breach of privacy of which a person is unaware is not recorded as such and triggers no response. Perceived breach of privacy that cannot be successfully counteracted, leads to stress and disturbance. A violation of privacy seems only permitted when it is for one's own good, for example, to get help, to achieve something, to get better and so on. Informed decision-making allows the individual to understand and, therefore, tolerate the invasion. The rationale has to outweigh the uncomfortable feelings or the intrusion can be unbearable. Signs of unsuccessful defence or regulation can be aggression or retreat, either psychological or physical. Abandoning an intended action, such as not giving a paper at a conference, not going to an interview, not going for a medical examination, is another form of retreat.

146

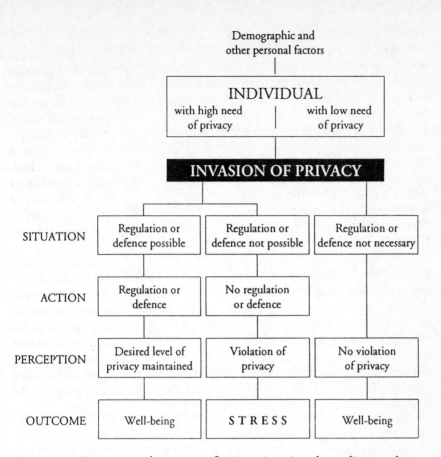

Figure 9.1   Reaction and outcome of privacy invasion depending on the
individual's constitution

This model shows the relationship between reaction to and outcome of privacy invasion depending on the individual's needs. Its most important feature is that individuals with a high need of privacy who are prevented from employing appropriate measures to maintain their desired level of privacy suffer from stress.

This theory is now open to being tested. One method would be to try to verify small portions of this theory, for example the concept of control in relationship to privacy, or underlying factors of privacy-regulating behaviour, in a specific substantive area, as proposed by Glaser and Strauss (1967). How far this theory can be applied to a background other than the German one should also be established. Another possibility is to additionally apply other formal theories on privacy and related areas and examine their mutual or distinct properties. This would give the theory derived from this study greater meaning. We use theories in an attempt to explain the relationships between observed phenomena, or as Dubin (1978) stated: 'the 'need' for theories lies in the human behaviour of wanting to impose order on unordered experiences' (p.6). By adding empirical knowledge to existing theories and modifying or reformulating them, they become more and more useful in their above mentioned function of explaining propositions that connect the concepts concerned. Therefore they enhance our understanding of our lived world. These theories could then be applied to different settings where they can be used to describe and explain phenomena and also to predict their outcome. Referring back to privacy, the existence of such a comprehensive theory could allow the development of strategies to prevent stressful invasions of a person's privacy, or the interpretation of observed outcome, for example inappropriate or incomprehensible behaviour, by connecting it with the cause, in this case invaded privacy. Unjust reactions based on ignorance would be diminished. One could then go further and develop models for practice which take into account the factors of privacy and its violation and provide, therefore, a more caring and therapeutic environment in the human interaction, wherever it may take place.

Summary

This chapter outlined a formal theory of privacy based on the substantive theory applied to the hospital context which was offered in the previous chapter. The propositions are tentative as they are based on primarily phenomenological data of this particular study. Nevertheless, the outlined theory could point to a direction in which a future theory might develop. The important relationship of privacy as a subjective feeling to the individual self was emphasized. Control was identified as the key factor in the perception of one's privacy. This feeling of control is maintained by negotiations and informed decision-making as to who gets the permission of access and to what degree. The first major issue that needs to be in the individual's control concerns exposure of identity and physical exposure. The second aspect is the access to one's territory and personal space. Thirdly, each potential intruder has to be assessed as to what his relationship is to the individual and, subsequently, how close this invader may be allowed. At the end of the chapter a model of reaction and outcome of privacy invasion depending on the individual's constitution was developed. Finally, testing of this theory is to be recommended.

10 Evaluation and recommendations

The last chapter of this book consists of a brief description of some important methodological aspects. It was felt that the researcher's personal experience should be outlined as well. This is important for the understanding why certain decisions have been made. It should also be of assistance to others undertaking replications of this study.

Methodological evaluation

Generally, the methods used and combined in this study seemed to be appropriate to achieve the aim of the research. Each method will be evaluated separately.

Interviews

Where the topic is all about an individual's perceptions, there is certainly no better way to elicit the desired responses than to use a phenomenological approach, and interviews as its means. At the beginning of the interview only a few patients could express any idea about privacy, and they were probably those who were better educated or verbally more versatile. But the opinion of people who did not have these attributes was sought as well. Therefore, semi-structured interviews that allow the researcher to rephrase and explain questions were most appropriate. It seems the right choice was made about the location of the data collection. If the respondents had been interviewed after discharge, one could argue that they would have felt more free to talk about their experiences. The danger of this approach is that memory fades once the setting is left behind and the outcome might be a too rosy picture of the patient's stay in hospital. French (1981) assumed that two factors – the patient's memory and the unpleasantness of the worry – seem to affect recall.

The analysis of the interviews posed the same problems as in a previous study by the same researcher (Bauer, 1991) because of the necessity to translate into a different language at one stage or another. To overcome this problem, every stage was cross-checked with the original transcripts to minimize distortion. After much reflection, the author would recommend that in future studies all analytical steps be performed in the original language of the interview and the results only then translated into the language of publication.

Questionnaire

The intention of the questionnaire was to examine if trends emerging from the interviews also applied to a larger sample. In so far as they allow access to a larger population and consume less time, questionnaires are justified. However, important methodological aspects emerged.

It transpired that the use of a questionnaire supports the 'everything is wonderful' mentality that patients so easily adopt when in hospital and dependent on the mercy of more powerful individuals. Based on their experience, Nehring and Geach (1973) warned against the use of written forms on patients because it was not a productive way of eliciting honest opinion. The responses in this study bear this out. When there were several items on one topic, the first question was generally answered in a more indifferent way, whereas the next questions, more detailed and concrete, provided different and even contradictory responses. There seems to be a danger in questionnaires of the respondents resorting to convenient non-demanding answers. It was felt to be justifiable to make the patients declare themselves. It seems that patients say more (and more honestly) in interviews than in questionnaires. A point of criticism might be that the patients who needed help in filling the forms may have been influenced by the presence of the researcher. The possible introduction of bias in face-to-face encounters is acknowledged. But questionnaires which were completed in private are not necessarily free of bias when we remember the patients' general uneasiness to give, for example, negative evidence about their stay in hospital. Interviews which do not risk personal influence on the interviewee by the interviewer would rarely be possible.

The Likert-type questionnaire used here moved away from the classical 'psychological trait summational scale' because of the vast topic with distinct areas (such as personal space, territoriality etc.). However, in future research the classical approach could be used for the different areas separately. The use of SPSS/PC+ for the analysis can be recommended for future similar research. Once mastered, it is a very straightforward and easy to use software package.

Rank-ordering

The rank-ordering procedure proved to be a simple but powerful method to elicit comparative judgement. Although subjective, ranking results seem to be more valid and reliable than those of the questionnaire because decisions have to be made in one way or another, whereas the questionnaire allows the respondent to be more indifferent. The analysis of the ranking turned out to be so easy and straightforward (manually as well as by computer) that the use of rank-ordering in the wide field of nursing research can only be recommended.

Other methodological issues
The study took place in a hospital with a large rural catchment area. Studies of patients in other areas of Germany with different cultural and social backgrounds and/or in major cities might yield different results.

Issues of validity have been discussed in the chapters on the different methods. Only a few comments shall be made here. The effect of the failure to achieve a full assessment of validity means that less confidence can be placed in the data. Due to time constraints, the sample size had to be kept manageable in both stages of the data collection. In the quantitative part of the study, a larger study population and a random sampling method would theoretically have enhanced the respresentativeness and, therefore, the general applicability of the findings. However, as this study aimed at understanding of an individual's experience, representativeness was not crucial. A validity check for qualitative data which is often recommended, is to go back to the respondents for validation of the analysed evidence. There are several problems with this approach. First of all, neither the patients nor the researcher were present long enough in the hospital setting to allow this kind of validation. A second problem is that over time memory fades, and this seems to apply particularly to patients after discharge from hospital. They might see things differently once they are in their own surroundings (selective memory). This, and the tendency of people to try to filter out the more negative aspects after some time, would invalidate the checks. A note should be added regarding the criticism of qualitative research and the oft-stated doubts as to its validity. What can be more valid than asking the person concerned about his, and exclusively his, experience? If we feel we cannot trust the respondent to express his feelings, we should not bother to ask him in the first place.

Retrospectively, if the study were to be conducted again, the interviews and the rank-ordering procedure would be employed again without any modification. If questionnaires were to be used, a very careful consideration of all aspects is necessary as well as a concentration on narrower topics that might allow a more detailed phrasing of the items. The possibility of evaluating the methods against each other demonstrates another beneficial aspect of method of triangulation.

Personal evaluation

When I started to approach patients I thought carefully about how to word the introduction of myself and the project. Considering the sensitivity of the topic, I started too cautiously and emphasized the voluntary nature of the participation so thoroughly that this (probably combined with their uneasiness at the prospect of giving critical evidence led many of the patients (similarly to Nehring and Geach, 1973) to refuse. This approach proved not to be very fruitful and I had only a limited period of time to complete the data collection. Very similar to Smith's (1992) personal experience, I changed to a more assertive way of introducing the study and I also stated its importance for future practice and emphasized the value of each patient's personal opinion. I assume that only after I had added that I was independent from the hospital but the management supported my work, did the recruitment of respondents become much more successful. How far this had manipulated the patients, is difficult to say. After around 100 patients it rather got on my nerves to repeat this invitation again and again and still sound convincing and enthusiastic. I had to remind myself that although I knew backwards what I was doing, the patient addressed was hearing it for the first time, and his participation depended on how I sold the idea. There was a conflict between allowing the patient the possibility of refusal and badly needing him to provide data. It was almost as if two people stood in front of him, one stressing the voluntary participation and protecting the subject's rights, the other begging silently: 'please, say yes'. There were some patients who agreed to participate in order to help me.

Before I had started the interviews I was very apprehensive about the outcome of these conversations. Would the patients say anything usable, and most important, would they tell me the 'truth'? The interviews turned out to be a very pleasant experience. Only occasionally was I slightly suspicious when elderly ladies tried to tell me they were not concerned about their privacy in hospital while their behaviour conveyed something quite different. I then remembered Colaizzi (1978) who stated that 'what is logically inexplicable may be existentially real and valid' (p.61). This could mean that those respondents employed unconsciously privacy protecting behaviour and they could rightfully state they had no problems because they consequently felt satisfied.

I also wondered how my being a nurse influenced responses. Would a retired teacher, an architect, a fellow patient or even a male nurse have evoked the same set of responses? However much I enjoyed talking to the patient, I often felt guilty: they wanted to talk, I wanted data. It soothed my conscience that the patients had a chance to reflect on their experience with somebody who wanted to listen. So in the end I could perhaps even have claimed to have done a good deed. What startled me was when the interview was over and I was happy with its rich data, patients thanked me for listening to them!

The dilemma of being a nurse and being a researcher is described by several authors (for example Malone, 1962). She stated 'the "nurse" in you may wish to deny responses which delight the researcher' (p.67), an experience I can only confirm. But it was not only the interviews that embarrassed me as a member of the nursing profession but the everyday observation of nursing routine. I recall just one particular incident. I was in a two-bed room asking one lady if she would like to participate in the study and we had a chat. A doctor entered the room and started to admit the newly arrived second patient. She had to get undressed and the physical examination started. Even as a nurse, I was not this patient's nurse. I felt I did not have the unwritten right to stay during this examination. I left the room although the doctor and nurses said I could stay. No one had asked the patient. Having had the patients' evidence in mind, I became even more sensitive concerning the patients' privacy than I had already been. It was not easy witnessing breaches of privacy while having no authority to intervene.

I was very pleased to perceive a great interest in the study from all sides. It seemed that my study had suddenly triggered an awareness of privacy which might have existed before but was firmly buried and, therefore, not talked about. It happened several times that I passed a group of patients and overheard them discussing the topic passionately. Patients, staff, even the 'Green Ladies' (volunteers who run errands and go shopping for the patients) asked where to get the findings and provided me providentially with their addresses to be informed about any publications. One patient even designed and developed a practicable screen for the patients' rooms which was about to go to a manufacturer when I left the hospital after my last data collection.

The whole project was very labour-intensive. The first part of the data collection and analysis ran smoothly as I employed a method I was familiar with. The second part proved to be more difficult and I had to turn to several people for advice. Armed with little theoretical knowledge about statistics and impeded by the use of a foreign language it proved difficult to follow all the statistical steps and to write up quantitative results. By far the most difficult part of the whole book, and this was again related to language problems, was the writing of the discussion. I felt it was not very demanding to interpret the data, but when I tried to raise these thoughts to a more abstract and theoretical level, I ran out of suitable vocabulary. After many unsuccessful attempts at inventing, constructing and manipulating the sentences, I was sometimes tempted to omit an idea altogether. During the entire course of this study, however, I enjoyed the work, the decisions, the 'brainwork', and at the end I had learned a lot from the process of investigating a topic of particular importance.

Recommendations

Further Research

There is a growing need to explore the concept of privacy in hospitals. This present study raised more questions than it answered. Following the inductive nature of this project, more data would have to be collected which could eventually be tested deductively. Similar studies in different hospitals with different catchment areas are as important as investigations of privacy in particular settings, such as Intensive Care Units, maternity wards, urological wards etc. The impact of current hospital design and ward environments on patients' privacy needs to be determined. Not enough is known about the way patients perceive their dependence while in hospital. Their perception of their territory, personal space, touch and other privacy-related concepts could only be treated superficially in this study. A possible change of the need for privacy as nurse and patient progress through the stages of their relationship has yet to be investigated. An identification and classification of patients' responses to invasions of privacy and their mechanisms to preserve privacy should be pursued.

Focusing on individuals other than patients, the visitors' perception of their privacy while visiting a patient is worthy of closer examination. Nurses' and doctors' attitudes towards patients' privacy are unknown at present, as is how far the consideration of patients' privacy influences their actions.

Only a few feasible approaches are suggested here. The possibilities are infinite.

Education, Management, Practice

'Adequate testing of conclusions derived from descriptive studies is necessary before direct application to practice should be made' (Gioiella, 1978:43). Taking this advice to heart, any recommendations based on the present study can only be tentative, and suggestive of the directions which might be adopted.

Although little is known about the patient's privacy, the general theoretical concepts of privacy, territoriality, personal space and related issues should be included in the nursing curriculum. 'Nursing, as a science, has a goal to understand those individuals being cared for in order to know how to care for them' (Lynch-Sauer, 1985:105-6). The aim should be to create an awareness of the problem, and to provide practical solutions as, for example, was attempted by Baumgart-Fütterer (1991). The role-model effect of ward sisters and staff nurses on student nurses should not be underestimated. The current findings highlighted a high demand for screens which can be utilized by the patient for individual purposes. It seems not to be premature to suggest the provision and consequently the actual use of appropriate screens. Before more research-based knowledge is available, it seems to be good advice to assume the patient we (and we means not only nurses but any health professional) care for is at least as sensitive towards his privacy as we are ourselves, and to act accordingly.

References

Aasterud, M. (1962), 'Defences against anxiety in the nurse-patient relationship', *Nursing Forum*, 1, 35-59.

Allekian, C. (1973), 'Intrusions of territory and personal space: an anxiety-inducing factor for hospitalized persons – an exploratory study', *Nursing Research*, 22, 3, 236-241.

Altman, I. (1975), *The Environment and Social Behavior. Privacy, Personal Space, Territory, Crowding*, Brooks/Cole, Monterey.

Altman, I. (1977), 'Privacy regulations: culturally universal or culturally specific?', *Journal of Social Issues*, 33, 3, 66-84.

Altman, I. and Chemers, M. (1980), *Culture and Environment*, Brooks/Cole, Monterey.

Altman, I. and Haythorn, W. (1967), 'The ecology of isolated groups', *Behavioral Science*, 12, 169-82.

Apsler, R. (1975), 'Effects of embarrassment on behavior toward others', *Journal of Personality and Social Psychology*, 32, 1, 145-53.

Archea, J. (1977), 'The place of architectural factors in behavioral theories of privacy', *Journal of Social Issues*, 33, 3, 116-37.

Ashenhurst, B. (1978), 'The privacy paradox', *The Lamp*, 35, 9, 32-5.

Barnett, K. (1972), 'A theoretical construct of the concepts of touch as they relate to nursing', *Nursing Research*, 21, 2, 102-10.

Barker, P. (1991), 'Questionnaire', in Cormack, D. (ed.), *The Research Process in Nursing*, Blackwell Scientific Publications, Oxford.

Barron, A. (1990), 'The right to personal space', *Nursing Times*, 86, 27, 28-32.

Bauer, I. (1991), *Nurses' and Patients' Perceptions of the First Hour of the Morning Shift in a Hospital in the Federal Republic of Germany*, Master Dissertation, University of Wales College of Medicine, Cardiff.

Baumgart-Fütterer, I. (1991), 'Umgang mit dem Schamgefühl der Patienten', *Krankenpflege-Journal*, 29, 7/8, 296-301.

Bates, A. (1964), 'Privacy – a useful concept?', *Social Forces*, 42, 429-34.

van den Berg, J. (1972a), *A Different Existence*, Duquesne University Press, Pittsburgh.

van den Berg, J. (1972b), *The Psychology of the Sickbed*, Humanities Press, New York.

Bloch, D. (1970), 'Privacy', in Carlson, C. (ed.), *Behavioral concepts and nursing intervention*, Lippincott, Philadelphia.

Bockmon, D. and Riemen, D. (1987), 'Qualitative versus quantitative nursing research', *Holistic Nursing Practice*, 2, 1, 71-5.

Boettcher, E. (1985), 'Boundary marking', *Journal of Psychosocial Nursing*, 23, 8, 25-30.

Bond, J. (1974), 'The construction of a scale to measure nurses' attitudes', *International Journal of Nursing Studies*, 11, 2, 75-84.

Brenner, M.; Brown, J. and Canter, D. (eds) (1985), *The Research Interview: uses and approaches*, Academic Press, London.

Brill, A. (1990), *Nobody's Business: Paradoxes of Privacy*, Addison-Wesley, Reading.

Brink, P. (1976), 'Critique of "Privacy and the hospitalization experience"', *Communicating Nursing Research*, 7, 172-80.

Brink, P. (1991), 'Issues of Reliability and Validity', in Morse, J. (ed.), *Qualitative Nursing Research, A Contemporary Dialogue*, Sage Publications, Newbury Park.

Bross, I. (1958), 'How to use Ridit analysis', *Biometrics*, 14,18-38.

Bryant, C. (1978), 'Privacy, Privatisation and Self-Determination', in Young, J. (ed.), *Privacy*, John Wiley and Sons, Chichester.

Bulmer, M. (ed.) (1982), *Social Research Ethics*, Macmillan, London.

Burch, R. (1989), 'On phenomenology and its practices', *Phenomenology and Pedagogy*, 7, 187-217.

Burgess, R. (1984), *In the Field. An Introduction to Field Research*, Unwin Hyman, London.

Burns, N. and Grove, S. (1987), *The Practice of Nursing Research*, Saunders, Philadelphia.

Burton, A. and Heller, L. (1964), 'The touching of the body', *The Psychoanalytic Review*, 51, 1, 122-34.

Buss, A. (1980), *Self-Consciousness and Social Anxiety*, W.H. Freeman & Company, San Francisco.

Buss, A.; Iscoe, I. and Buss, E. (1979), 'The development of embarrassment', *The Journal of Psychology*, 103, 227-30.

Canter, D. (1984), 'The Environmental Context of Nursing: Looking Beyond the Ward', in Skevington, S. (ed.), *Understanding Nurses; The Social Psychology of Nursing*, John Wiley & Sons, Chichester.

Canter, S. and Canter, D. (1979), 'Building for Therapy', in Canter, D. and Canter, S. (eds), *Designing for Therapeutic Environments. A Review of Research*, John Wiley & Sons, Chichester.

Cantrell, T. (1978), 'Privacy – The Medical Problems', in Young, J. (ed.), *Privacy*, John Wiley & Sons, Chichester.

Cartwright, A. (1964), *Human Relations and Hospital Care*, Routledges & Kegan Paul, London.

Cavallin, B. and Houston, B. (1980), 'Aggressiveness, maladjustment, body experience and the protective function of personal space', *Journal of Clinical Psychology*, 36, 1, 170-76.

Cavan, S. (1977), Review of Douglas, J. (1976) *Investigative Social Research*, *American Journal of Sociology*, 83, 809-11.

Chesla, C. (1992), 'When qualitative and quantitative findings do not converge', *Western Journal of Nursing Research*, 14, 5, 681-5.

Clade, H. (1989), 'Langzeitstudie der Meinungsforscher: "Die Krankenhäuser sind besser als ihr Ruf"', *Krankenhaus Umschau*, 58, 6, 488-96.

Cohen, M. (1987), 'A historical overview of the phenomenologic movement', *IMAGE: Journal of Nursing Scholarship*, 19, 1, 31-4.

Colaizzi, P. (1978), 'Psychological Research as the Phenomenologist Views It', in Valle, R. and King, M. (eds), *Existential-phenomenological alternatives for psychology*, Oxford University Press, New York.

Conover, W. (1980), *Practical Nonparametric Statistics*, John Wiley & Sons, New York.

Cooper, K. (1984), 'Territorial behavior among the institutionalized. A nursing perspective', *Journal of Psychosocial Nursing*, 22, 12, 6-11.

Counsel and Care (1991), *Not Such Private Places*, Councel and Care, London.

Cowles, K. (1988), 'Issues in qualitative research on sensitive topics', *Western Journal of Nursing Research*, 10, 2, 163-79.

Crano, W. and Brewer, M. (1986), *Principles and Methods of Social Research*, Allyn and Bacon, Boston.

Creighton, H. (1985), 'Right of privacy: Limit', *Nursing Management*, 16, 3, 15-7.

Davidson, L. (1990), 'A room of their own?', *Nursing Times*, 86, 27, 32-3.

Davis, A. (1978), 'The Phenomenological Approach in Nursing Research', in Chaska, N. (ed.), *The Nursing Profession. Views through the Mist*, McGraw-Hill, New York.

Davis, J. (1984), 'Don't Fence Me In', *American Journal of Nursing*, 84, 9, 1141, 1143.

Dean, J. and Whyte, W. (1958), '"How do you know if the informant is telling the truth?"', *Human Organization*, 17, 2, 34-8.

De Augustinis, J.; Isani, R. and Kumler, F. (1963), 'Ward Study: The Meaning of Touch in Interpersonal Communication', in Burd, S. and Marshall, M. (eds), *Some Clinical Approaches to Psychiatric Nursing*, Macmillan, New York.

Denzin, N. (1978), *The Research Act*, McGraw-Hill, New York.

Denzin, N. (1989), *Interpretive Interactionism*, Sage Publications, Newbury Park.

Dobson, S. (1991), *Transcultural Nursing*, Scutari Press, London.

Dubin, R. (1978), *Theory Building*, The Free Press, Macmillan, New York.

Duffy, M. (1987), 'Methodological triangulation: a vehicle for merging quantitative and qualitative research methods', *IMAGE: Journal of Nursing Scholarship*, 19, 3, 130-3.

Duke, M. and Novicki, S. (1972), 'A new measure and social-learning model for interpersonal distance', *Journal of Experimental Research in Personality*, 6, 119-32.

Durr, C. (1971), 'Hands that help ... But how?', *Nursing Forum*, 10, 4, 392-400.

Edelmann, R. (1981), 'Embarrassment: the state of research', *Current Psychological Reviews*, 1, 125-37.

Edelmann, R. (1985), 'Social embarrassment: an analysis of the process', *Journal of Social and Personal Relationships*, 2, 195-213.

Edelmann, R. and Hampson, S. (1979), 'Changes in non-verbal behaviour during embarrassment', *British Journal of Social and Clinical Psychology*, 18, 385-90.

Edwards, A. (1957), *Techniques of Attitude Scale Construction*, Appleton-Century-Crofts, New York.

Elliott, J. (1982), *Living in Hospital*, King Edward's Hospital Fund for London.

Emerson, J. (1973), 'Behavior in Private Places: Sustaining Definitions of Reality in Gynecological Examinations', in Wertz, R. (ed.), *Readings on Ethical and Social Issues in Biomedicine*, Prentice-Hall, Englewood Cliffs.

English, J. and Morse, J. (1988), 'The 'difficult' elderly patient: adjustment or maladjustment?', *International Journal of Nursing Studies*, 25, 1, 23-39.

Ernst, M. and Schwartz, A. (1962), *Privacy, The Right to Be Let Alone*, Macmillan, New York.

Esser, A.; Chamberlain, A.; Chapple, E. and Kline, N. (1965), 'Territoriality of patients on a research ward', *Recent Advances in Biological Psychiatry*, 7, 37-44.

Etzioni, A. (1968), 'Basic human needs, alienation and inauthenticity', *American Sociological Review*, 33, 6, 870-85.

Evans, G. and Howard, R. (1973), 'Personal space', *Psychological Bulletin*, 80, 4, 334-344.

Fawcett, J. and Downs, F. (1992), *The Relationship of Theory and Research*, F. A. Davis, Philadelphia.

Felipe, N. and Sommer, R. (1966), 'Invasions of personal space', *Social Problems*, 14, 2, 206-14.

Field, P. (1981), 'A phenomenological look at giving an injection', *Journal of Advanced Nursing*, 6, 291-96.

Field, P. and Morse, J. (1985), *Nursing Research: The Application of Qualitative Approaches*, Croom Helm, London.

Fielding, N. and Fielding, J. (1986), *Linking Data*, Sage Publications, Beverly Hills.

Fields, C. (1977), 'A growing problem for researchers: protecting privacy', *The Chronicle of Higher Education*, 14, 10, 1 and 15.

Fischer, C. (1971), 'Toward the Structure of Privacy: Implications for Psychological Assessment', in Giorgi, A.; Fischer, W. and von Ekartsberg, R. (eds), *Duquesne Studies in Phenomenological Psychology, Volume I*, Duquesne University Press, Pittsburgh.

Fleiss, J. (1981), *Statistical Methods for Rates and Proportions*, Wiley & Sons, New York.

Foster, J. (1992), *Starting SPSS/PC+. A beginner's guide to data analysis*, Sigma Press, Wilmslow.

Freidson, E. (1970), *Profession of Medicine*, Dodd, Mead & Company, New York.

French, K. (1979), 'Some Anxieties of Elective Surgery Patients and the Desire for Reassurance and Information', in Oborne, D.; Gruneberg, M. and Eiser, J. (eds), *Research in Psychology and Medicine, Volume II*, Academic Press, London.

French, K. (1981), 'Methodological considerations in hospital patient opinion surveys', *International Journal of Nursing Studies*, 18, 1, 7-32.

Freud, S. (1960), *Group Psychology and the Analysis of the Ego*, Bantam Books, New York.

Friedman, M. (1937), 'The use of ranks to avoid the assumption of normality implicit in the analysis of variance', *Journal of the American Statistical Association*, 32, 675-701.

Frude, N. (1987), *A Guide to SPSS/PC+*, Macmillan Education, Basingstoke.

Gainsborough, H. (1970), 'Privacy and patient care', *British Hospital Journal and Social Service Review*, April 24, 751-52.

Geden, E. and Begeman, A. (1981), 'Personal preferences of hospitalized adults', *Research in Nursing and Health*, 4, 2, 237-41.

George, J. and Quattrone, M. (1985), 'Search for patient identification: An invasion of privacy?', *Journal of Emergency Nursing*, 11, 6, 335-36.

Gifford, R. (1987), *Environmental Psychology, Principles and Practice*, Allyn and Bacon, Boston.

Giger, J. and Davidhizar, R. (1990), 'Culture and space', *Advancing Clinical Care*, 5, 6, 8-11.

Gioiella, E. (1978), 'The relationships between slowness of response, state anxiety, social isolation and self-esteem, and preferred personal space in the elderly', *Journal of Gerontological Nursing*, 4, 1, 40-3.

Giorgi, A. (1975), 'An application of phenomenological method in psychology', *Duquesne Studies in Phenomenological Psychology*, 2, 82-103.

Giorgi, A. (1986), 'Theoretical Justification for the Use of Descriptions in Psychological Research', in Ashworth, P.; Giorgi, A. and de Koning, A. (eds), *Qualitative Research in Psychology*, Duquesne University Press, Pittsburgh.

Glaser, B. and Strauss, A. (1967), *The Discovery of Grounded Theory: strategies for qualitative research*, Aldine de Gruyter, New York.

Globig, K.-F. (1991), 'Das humane Krankenhaus als Verwaltungsaufgabe', *Krankenhaus Umschau*, 60, 4, 275-86.

Goffman, E. (1959), *The Presentation of Self in Everyday Life*, Pelican Books, London.

Goffman, E. (1961), *Asylums*, Peregrine Books, London.

Goffman, E. (1963), *Behavior in public places: notes on the social organization of gatherings*, The Free Press of Glencoe, New York.

Goffman, E. (1971), *Relations in Public*, Basic Books, New York.

Goodwin, L. and Goodwin, W. (1984), 'Qualitative vs. Quantitative research or qualitative *and* quantitative research?', *Nursing Research*, 33, 6, 378-80.

Guilford, J. (1954), *Psychometric Methods*, McGraw-Hill, New York.

Hackworth, J. (1976), 'Relationship between spatial density and sensory overload, personal space, and systolic and diastolic blood pressure', *Perceptual and Motor Skills*, 43, 867-72.

Hagan, T. (1986), 'Interviewing the Downtrodden', in Ashworth, P.; Giorgi, A. and de Koning, A. (eds), *Qualitative Research in Psychology*, Duquesne University Press, Pittsburgh.

Hall, E. (1959), *The Silent Language*, Doubleday, New York.

Hall, E. (1966), *The Hidden Dimension*, The Bodley Head, London.

Hall, E. and Whyte, W. (1976), 'Intercultural Communication: A Guide to Men of Action', in Brink, P. (ed.), *Transcultural Nursing. A Book of Readings*, Prentice- Hall, Englewood Cliffs.

Hays, W. (1973), *Statistics for the Social Sciences*, Holt, Rinehart & Winston, London.

Hayter, J. (1981), 'Territoriality as a universal need', *Journal of Advanced Nursing*, 6, 79-85.

Heidegger, M. (1929), *Sein und Zeit*, Niemeyer, Halle a.d.S.

Heidt, P. (1981), 'Effect of therapeutic touch on anxiety level of hospitalized patients', *Nursing Research*, 30, 1, 32-7.

Heidt, P. (1991), 'Helping patients to rest: Clinical studies in therapeutic touch', *Holistic Nursing Practice*, 5, 4, 57-66.

Helber, A. (1991), 'Der "schwierige" Patient', *Deutsche Krankenpflegezeitschrift*, 44, 10, 733-37.

Hinchliff, S. (1986), *Teaching Clinical Nursing*, Churchill Livingstone, Edinburgh.

Hockey, L. (1991), 'The Nature of Research', in Cormack, D. (ed.), *The Research Process in Nursing*, Blackwell Scientific Publications, Oxford.

Hodgson, H. (1975), 'Patients and privacy', *The Hospital and Health Service Review*, 1971, 44-6.

Holahan, C. and Wandersman, A. (1987), 'The Community Psychology Perspective in Environmental Psychology', in Stokol, D. and Altman, I. (eds), *Handbook of Environmental Psychology, Volume I and II*, John Wiley & Sons, New York.

Horowitz, M. (1965), 'Human spatial behavior', *American Journal of Psychotherapy*, 19, 20-8.

Hubeli, E. (1989), 'Das andere Krankenzimmer', *Werk, Bauen + Wohnen*, 43, 4, 4-8.

Husserl, E. (1976), 'Ideen zu einer reinen Phänomenologie und phänomenologischen Philosophie. Erster Band. Allgemeine Einführung in die reine Phänomenologie', in Schuhmann, K. (ed.), *Husserliana Band III/1*, Martinus Nijhoff, Den Haag.

Hutchinson, S. and Wilson, H. (1992), 'Validity threats in scheduled semi-structured research interviews', *Nursing Research*, 41, 2, 117-9.

Hycner, R. (1985), 'Some guidelines for the phenomenological analysis of interview data', *Human Studies*, 8, 279-303.

Ingham, R. (1987), 'Privacy and Psychology', in Young, J. (ed.), *Privacy*, John Wiley & Sons, Chichester.

Jaco, E. (1979), *Patients, Physicians and Illness. A Scourcebook in Behavioural Science and Health*, The Free Press, London.

Jick, T. (1979), 'Mixing qualitative and quantitative methods: triangulation in action', *Administrative Science Quarterly*, 24, 602-11.

Johnson, F. (1979), 'Response to territorial intrusion by nursing home residents', *Advances in Nursing Science*, 1, 4, 21-34.

Johnston, J. (1988), 'Preserving privacy and confidentiality for the emergency patient', *Emergency Nursing Reports*, 3, 4, 1-8.

Jones, E. and Kay, M. (1992), 'Instrumentation in cross-cultural research', *Nursing Research*, 41, 3, 186-8.

Juchli, L. (1991), *Krankenpflege*, Thieme, Stuttgart.

van Kaam, A. (1959), 'Phenomenal analysis: exemplified by a study of the experience of "really feeling understood"', *Journal of Individual Psychology*, 15, 66-72.

van Kaam, A. (1969), *Existential Foundation of Psychology*, Doubleday, New York.

Kelly, M. and May, D. (1982), 'Good and bad patients: a review of the literature and a theoretical critique', *Journal of Advanced Nursing*, 7, 147-56.

Kenny, C. and Canter, D. (1979), 'Evaluating Acute General Hospitals', in Canter, D. and Canter, S. (eds), *Designing for Therapeutic Environments. A Review of Research*, John Wiley & Sons, Chichester.

Kerlinger, F. (1986), *Foundations of Behavioral Research*, CBS Publishing Japan Ltd, New York.

Kerr, J. (1982), 'An overview of theory and research related to space use in hospitals', *Western Journal of Nursing Research*, 4, 4, 395-405.

Kerr, J. (1985), 'Space use, privacy, and territoriality', *Western Journal of Nursing Research*, 7, 2, 199-219.

Kidder, L. and Judd, C. (1986), *Research Methods in Social Relations*, CSB Publishing Japan Ltd., New York.

Knaak, P. (1984), 'Phenomenological research', *Western Journal of Nursing Research*, 6, 1, 107-14.

Knafl, K. and Howard, M. (1984), 'Interpreting and reporting qualitative research', *Research in Nursing and Health*, 7, 17-24.

Kornfeld, D. (1977), 'The Hospital Environment: Its Impact on the Patient', in Moos, R. (ed.), *Coping with physical illness*, Plenum, New York.

Kvale, S. (1983), 'The qualitative research interview: a phenomenological and a hermeneutical mode of understanding', *Journal of Phenomenological Psychology*, 14, 2, 171-96.

Lane, P. (1989), 'Nurse-client perceptions: the double standard of touch', *Issues in Mental Health Nursing*, 10, 1, 1-13.

Lange, S. (1970), 'Shame', in Carlson, C. (ed.), *Behavioral Concepts and Nursing Intervention*, Lippincott, Philadelphia.

Laufer, R. and Wolfe, M. (1977), 'Privacy as a concept and a social issue: a multidimensional developmental theory', *Journal of Social Issues*, 33, 3, 22-42.

Lawler, J. (1991), *Behind the Screens*, Churchill Livingstone, Melbourne.

Lazarus, R. (1966), *Psychological stress and the coping process*, McGraw Hill, New York.

LeCompte, M. and Goetz, J. (1982), 'Problems of reliability and validity in ethnographic research', *Review of Educational Research*, 52, 1, 31-60.

Lee, D. (1959), *Freedom and Culture*, Prentice-Hall, Englewood Cliffs.

Leininger, M. (1985), *Qualitative Research Methods in Nursing*, Grune and Stratton, Orlando.

Levine, M. (1968), 'Knock before entering the personal space bubbles – Part II', *CHART*, 65, 82-4.

Likert, R. (1932), *A Technique for the Measurement of Attitudes*, Archives of Psychology (No. 140), Columbia University Press, New York.

Little, K. (1965), 'Personal space', *Journal of Experimental Social Psychology*, 1, 3, 237-47.

Locsin, A. (1984), 'The concept of touch', *Philippine Journal of Nursing*, 54, 4, 114-23,140.

Lofland, J. and Lofland, L. (1984), *Analyzing social settings: a guide to qualitative observation and analysis*, Wadsworth, Belmont.

Long, G. (1984), 'Psychological tension and closeness to others: stress and interpersonal distance preference', *The Journal of Psychology*, 117, 143-6.

Lorber, J. (1979), 'Good Patients and Problem Patients: Conformity and Deviance in a General Hospital', in Jaco, E. (ed.), *Patients, Physicians, and Illness*, The Free Press, New York.

Lorensen, M. (1983), 'Effects of Touch in Patients during a Crisis Situation in Hospital', in Wilson-Barnett, J. (ed.), *Nursing Research,* John Wiley & Sons, Chichester.

Louis, M. (1981), 'Personal space boundary needs of elderly persons: an empirical study', *Journal of Gerontological Nursing*, 7, 7, 395-400.

Lyman, S. and Scott, M. (1967), 'Territoriality: a neglected sociological dimension', *Social Problems*, 15, 2, 236-49.

Lynch-Sauer, J. (1985), 'Using a Phenomenological Research Method to Study Nursing Phenomena', in Leininger, M. (ed.), *Qualitative Research Methods in Nursing*, Grune and Stratton, Orlando.

162

MacCormick, D. (1974), 'Privacy: a problem of definition?', *British Journal of Law and Society*, 1, 1, 75-8.

MacGregor, F. (1967), 'Uncooperative patients: some cultural interpretations', *American Journal of Nursing*, 67, 1, 88-91.

Mallon-Palmer, M. (1980), 'Personal space theories: lessons for nurses', *The Australian Nurses' Journal*, 10, 5, 36-8.

van Manen, M. (1990), *Researching Lived Experience. Human Science for an Action Sensitive Pedagogy*, The Althouse Press, Ontario.

Marshall, C. and Rossman, G. (1989), *Designing Qualitative Research*, Sage Publications, Newbury Park.

Marx, M.; Werner, P. and Cohen-Mansfield, J. (1989), 'Agitation and touch in the nursing home', *Psychological Reports*, 64, 1019-26.

McBride, G.; King, M. and James, J. (1965), 'Social proximity effects on galvanic skin responses in adult humans', *The Journal of Psychology*, 61, 153-7.

McCloskey, H. (1971), 'The political ideal of privacy', *Philosophical Quarterly*, 21, 303-14.

McDowell, I. and Newell, C. (1987), *Measuring Health: A Guide to Rating Scales and Questionnaires*, Oxford University Press, New York.

McElroy, J. and Middlemist, R. (1983), 'Personal space, crowding, and the interference model of test anxiety', *Psychological Reports*, 53, 2, 419-24.

McGuire, M. and Polsky, R. (1983), 'Sociospatial behavioral relationships among hospitalized psychiatric patients', *Psychiatry Research*, 8, 3, 225-36.

McLaughlin, F. and Marascuilo, L. (1990), *Advanced Nursing and Health Care Research*, W.B. Saunders, Philadelphia.

Mead, G. (1934), *Mind, Self, and Society*, The University of Chicago Press, Chicago.

Meijer, M. (1992), *Nurses' view on the general hospital nursing environment*, Master-Dissertation, University of Wales College of Medicine, Cardiff.

Meisenhelder, J. (1982), 'Boundaries of personal space', *Image*, 14, 1, 16-9.

Menzies, I. (1970), *The Functioning of Social Systems as a Defence Against Anxiety*, Tavistock, London.

Mercer, L. (1966), 'Touch: comfort or threat?', *Perspectives in Psychiatric Care*, 4, 3, 20-5.

Merleau-Ponty, M. (1962), *The Phenomenology of Perception*, Routledge & Kegan Paul, London.

Merry, S. (1981), 'Defensible space undefended. Social factors in crime control through environmental design', *Urban Affairs Quarterly*, 16, 4, 397-422.

Milligan, M. (1987), 'When the lack of privacy gets to your patient', *RN*, 50, 3, 17-18.

Minckley, B. (1968), 'Space and place in patient care', *American Journal of Nursing*, 68, 3, 510-6.

Morgan, C. (1986), 'Ensuring dignity and self esteem for patients and clients', *The Professional Nurse*, 2, 1, 12-4.

Morse, J. (1991), *Qualitative Nursing Research. A Contemporary Dialogue*, Sage Publications, Newbury Park.

Moser, C. and Kalton, G. (1971), *Survey Methods in Social Investigation*, Heinemann Educational Books, London.

Mulaik, J.; Megenity, J.; Cannon, R.; Chance, K; Cannella, K.; Garland, L. and Gilead, M. (1991), 'Patients' perceptions of nurses' use of touch', *Western Journal of Nursing Research*, 13, 3, 306-23.

Munhall, P. and Oiler, C. (eds) (1986), *Nursing Research, A Qualitative Perspective*, Appleton-Century-Crofts, Norwalk.

Nehring, V. and Geach, B. (1973), 'Patients' evaluation of their care. Why they don't complain', *Nursing Outlook*, 21, 5, 317-21.

Nelson, M. and Paluck, R. (1980), 'Territorial markings, self-concept, and mental status of the institutionalized elderly', *The Gerontologist*, 20, 1, 96-8.

Neufert, E. (1979), *Bauentwurfslehre*, Vieweg & Sohn, Braunschweig.

Nieswiadomy, R. (1987), *Foundations of Nursing Research*, Appleton/Lange, Norwalk.

Norusis, M. (1988), *The SPSS guide to data analysis for SPSS/PC+*, SPSS, Chicago.

Nuffield Provincial Hospital Trusts (1955), *Studies in the Functions and Design of Hospitals*, Oxford University Press, London.

Nunnally, J. (1978), *Psychometric Theory*, McGraw-Hill, New York.

Oiler, C. (1982), 'The phenomenological approach in nursing research', *Nursing Research*, 31, 3, 178-81.

Oiler, C. (1986), 'Phenomenology: The Method', in Munhall, P. and Oiler, C. (eds), *Nursing Research: A Qualitative Perspective*, Appleton-Century-Crofts, Norwalk.

Oland, L. (1978), 'The Need for Territoriality', in Yura, H. and Walsh, M. (eds), *Human Needs and the Nursing Process*, Appleton-Century-Crofts, New York.

Oliver, S. and Redfern S. (1991), 'Interpersonal communication between nurses and elderly patients: refinement of an observation schedule', *Journal of Advanced Nursing*, 16, 30-8.

Omery, A. (1983), 'Phenomenology: a method for nursing research', *Advances in Nursing Science*, 5, 2, 49-63.

O'Neal, E.; Brunault, M.; Marquis, J. and Carifio, M. (1979), 'Anger and the body- buffer zone', *The Journal of Social Psychology*, 108, 135-6.

Oppenheim, A. (1992), *Questionnaire Design, Interviewing and Attitude Measurement*, Pinter, London.

Pallikkathayil, L. and Morgan, S. (1991), 'Phenomenology as a method for conducting clinical research', *Applied Nursing Research*, 4, 4, 195-200.

Pan American Health Organization (1983), 'Quantitative and qualitative methods: a choice or a combination?', *Epidemiological Bulletin*, 4, 2, 12-3.

Parse, R.; Coyne, A. and Smith, M. (1985), *Nursing Research. Qualitative Methods*, Brady Communications Comp, Bowie, Maryland.

Parsons, T. (1951), *The Social System*, Routledge & Kegan Paul, London.

Phillips, J. (1979), 'An exploration of perception of body boundary, personal space, and body size in elderly persons', *Perceptual and Motor Skills*, 48, 1, 299-308.

Pluckhan, M. (1968), 'SPACE: The silent language', *Nursing Forum*, 7, 4, 386-97.

Polit, D. and Hungler, B. (1987), *Nursing Research, Principles and Methods*, Lippincott, Philadelphia.

Polit, D. and Hungler, B. (1989), *Essentials of Nursing Research*, Lippincott, Philadelphia.

Polkinghorne, D. (1989), 'Phenomenological Research Methods', in Valle, R. and Halling, S. (eds), *Existential-phenomenological Perspectives in Psychology*, Plenum, New York.

Pomeroy, W. (1963), 'The reluctant respondent', *Public Opinion Quarterly*, 27, 287- 93.

Prescott, P. and Soeken, K. (1989), 'The potential uses of pilot work', *Nursing Research*, 38, 1, 60-2.

Price, D. and Barrell, J. (1980), 'An experiential approach with quantitative methods: a research paradigm', *Journal of Humanistic Psychology*, 20, 3, 75-95.

Ramos, M. (1989), 'Some ethical implications of qualitative research', *Research in Nursing and Health*, 12, 1, 57-63.

Raphael, W. (1973), *Patients and Their Hospitals*, King Edward's Hospital Fund for London.

Raphael, W. (1974), *Just an Ordinary Patient*, King Edward's Hospital Fund for London.

Raphael, W. (1979), *Old people in hospital*, King Edward's Hospital Fund for London.

Raphael, W. and Peers, V. (1972), *Psychiatric Hospitals Viewed by Their Patients*, King Edward's Hospital Fund, London.

Rawnsley, M. (1980), 'The concept of privacy', *Advances in Nursing Science*, 2, 2, 25-31.

Reid, F. (1976), 'Space, territory and psychiatry', *Mental Health and Society*, 3, 77-91.

Reinharz, S. (1983), 'Phenomenology as a dynamic process', *Phenomenology and Pedagogy*, 1, 77-9.

Reizenstein, J. (1982), 'Hospital Design and Human Behavior: a Review of the Recent Literature', in Baum, A. and Singer, J. (eds), *Advances in Environmental Psychology: Volume 4. Environment and Health*, Erlbaum, Hillsdale.

Riemen, D. (1986), 'The Essential Structure of a Caring Interaction: Doing Phenomenology', in Munhall, P. and Oiler, C. (eds), *Nursing Research: A Qualitative Perspective*, Appleton-Century-Crofts, Norwalk.

Ritter, J. (ed.) (1972), *Historisches Wörterbuch der Philosophie*, Schwabe, Basel/Stuttgart.

Ritter, S. and von Eiff, W. (1988), *Krankenhaussanierung*, Ecomed, Landsberg.

Roberts, J. and Gregor, T. (1971), 'Privacy: A Cultural View', in Pennock, J. and Chapman, J. (eds), *Privacy*, Atherton Press, New York.

Roberts, S. (1986), *Behavioral Concepts and the Critically Ill Patient*, Appleton-Century-Crofts, Norwalk.

Robinson, L. (1979), 'A therapeutic paradox – to support intimacy and regression or privacy and autonomy', *Journal of Psychiatric Nursing*, 17, 10, 19-23.

Roosa, W. (1982), 'Territory and privacy. Residents' views: findings of a survey', *Geriatric Nursing*, 3, 4, 241-3.

Roper, N.; Logan, W. and Tierney, A. (1990), *The Elements of Nursing*, Churchill Livingstone, Edinburgh.

Rosenbaum, J. (1988), 'Validity in qualitative research', *Nursing Papers/Perspectives en nursing*, 19, 3, 55-66.

Rosengren, W. and DeVault, S. (1963), 'The Sociology of Time and Space in an Obstetrical Hospital', in Freidson, E. (ed.), *The Hospital in Modern Society*, The Free Press, New York.

Rosenhan, D. (1973), 'On being sane in insane places', *Science*, 179, 250-8.

Rosnow, R. and Rosenthal, R. (1970), 'Volunteer Effects in Behavioral Research', in Newcomb, T. (ed.), *New Directions in Psychology, Volume 4*, Holt & Rinehart, Englewood Cliffs .

Royal Commission on the National Health Service (1979), *Report*, Her Majesty's Stationery Office, London.

Salsberry, P. (1989), 'Phenomenological research in nursing. Commentary: fundamental issues', *Nursing Science Quarterly*, 2, 1, 9-13.

Sarosi, G. (1968), 'A critical theory: the nurse as a fully human person', *Nursing Forum*, 7, 4, 349-64.

Sartre, J.-P. (1943), *L' être et le néant. Essai d'ontologie phénoménologique*, Gallimard, Paris.

Schatzman, L. and Strauss, A. (1973), *Field Research; Strategies for a Natural Sociology*, Prentice-Hall, Englewood Cliffs.

Schultz, E. (1977), 'Privacy: the forgotten need', *The Canadian Nurse*, 73, 7, 33-4.

Schuster, E. (1976a), 'Privacy and the hospitalization experience', *Communicating Nursing Research*, 7, 153-71.

Schuster, E. (1976b), 'Privacy, the patient and hospitalization', *Social Science and Medicine*, 10, 245-8.

Schutz, A. (1970), *On Phenomenology and Social Relations*, University of Chicago Press, Chicago.

Schwartz, B. (1968), 'The social psychology of privacy', *The American Journal of Sociology*, 73, 741-52.

Sebba, R. and Churchman, A. (1983), 'Territories and territoriality in the home', *Environment and Behavior*, 15, 2, 191-210.

Seelye, A. (1982). 'Hospital ward layout and nurse staffing', *Journal of Advanced Nursing*, 7, 195-201.

Seligman, M. (1975), *Helplessness. On Depression, Development and Death*, W.H. Freeman and Company, San Francisco.

Shields, P.; Morrison, P. and Hart, D. (1988), 'Consumer satisfaction on a psychiatric ward', *Journal of Advanced Nursing*, 13, 396-400.

Shumaker, S. and Reizenstein, J. (1982), 'Environmental Factors Affecting Inpatient Stress in Acute Care Hospitals', in Evans, G. (ed.), *Environmental Stress*, Cambridge University Press, New York.

Slocumb, E. and Cole, F. (1991), 'A practical approach to content validation', *Applied Nursing Research*, 4, 4, 192-5.

Smith, B. and Cantrell, P. (1988), 'Distance in nurse-patient encounters', *Journal of Psychosocial Nursing*, 26, 2, 22-6.

Smith, H. (1981), *Strategies of Social Research*, Prentice-Hall, Englewood Cliffs.

Smith, L. (1992), 'Ethical issues in interviewing', *Journal of Advanced Nursing*, 17, 1, 98-103.

Sommer, B. and Sommer, R. (1991), *A Practical Guide To Behavioral Research*, Oxford University Press, New York.

Sommer, R. (1959), 'Studies in personal space', *Sociometry*, 22, 247-60.

Sommer, R. (1969), *Personal Space: The Behavioral Basis of Design*, Prentice-Hall, Englewood Cliffs.

Sommer, R. and Dewar, R. (1963), 'The Physical Environment of the Ward', in Freidson, E. (ed.), *The Hospital in Modern Society*, The Free Press, New York.

Spiegelberg, H. (1982), *The Phenomenological Movement. A Historical Introduction*, Martinus Nijhoff Publishers, The Hague.

Spinelli, E. (1989), *The Interpreted World. An Introduction to Phenomenological Psychology*, Sage Publications, London.

Stockwell, F. (1984), *The Unpopular Patient*, Croom Helm, London.

Stratton, J. (1981), *Personal Space Preferences of Hospital Children for Nurses, Doctors, Family Members and Strangers*, University of Missouri, Columbia.

Sundstrom, E. and Altman, I. (1974), 'Field study of territorial behavior and dominance', *Journal of Personality and Social Psychology*, 30, 1, 115-24.

Sundstrom, E. and Altman, I. (1976), 'Interpersonal relationships and personal space: research review and theoretical model', *Human Ecology*, 4, 1, 47-67.

Sundstrom, E.; Herbert, R. and Brown, D. (1982), 'Privacy and communication in an open-plan office: A case study', *Environment and Behavior*, 14, 379-92.

Swanson-Kauffman, K. and Schonwald, E. (1988), 'Phenomenology', in Sarter, B. (ed.), *Paths to Knowledge. Innovative Research Methods for Nursing*, National League for Nursing, New York.

Tate, J. (1980), 'The need for personal space in institutions for the elderly', *Journal of Gerontological Nursing*, 6, 8, 439-49.

Taylor, S. and Bogdan, R. (1984), *Introduction to qualitative research methods: the search for meanings*, John Wiley and Sons, New York.

Thayer, S. (1988), 'Close encounters', *Psychology Today*, March, 31-6.

Thorndike, R. (1963), 'Reliability', in Anastasi, A. (1966) (ed.), *Testing Problems in Perspective*, American Council on Education, Washington.

Treece, E. and Treece, J. (1986), *Elements of Research in Nursing*, C.V. Mosby Company, St. Louis.

Trierweiler, R. (1978), 'Personal Space and its effects on an elderly individual in a long-term care institution', *Journal of Gerontological Nursing*, 4, 5, 21-3.

Tungpalan, L. (1982), 'Proxemics and the nurse', *Academy of Nursing of the Philippines Papers*, 17, 1-2, 12-7.

Valle, R.; King, M. and Halling, S. (1989), 'An Introduction to Existential-Phenomenological Thought in Psychology', in Valle, R. and Halling, S. (eds), *Existential-Phenomenological Perspectives in Psychology*, Plenum Press, New York.

Velecky, L. (1978), 'The Concept of Privacy', in Young, J. (ed.), *Privacy*, John Wiley & Sons, Chichester.

Viguers, R. (1959), 'Be kind to "impossible" patients – they're scared', *The Modern Hospital*, 92, 1, 70-1.

Visotsky, H; Hamburg, D.; Goss, M. and Lebovits, B. (1961), 'Coping behavior under extreme stress', *Archives of General Psychiatry*, 5, 423-48.

Vousden, M. (1987), 'Private Lives', *Nursing Times*, 83, 24, 41-3.

Wainwright, P. (1985), 'Impact of Hospital Architecture on the Patient in Pain', in Copp, L. (ed.), *Perspectives on Pain*, Churchill Livingstone, Edinburgh.

Waltz, C.; Strickland, O. and Lenz, E. (1991), *Measurement in Nursing Research*, F. A. Davis Company, Philadelphia.

Warren, S. and Brandeis, L. (1890), 'The right to privacy', *Harvard Law Review*, 4, 5, 193-220.

Weiss, S. (1979), 'The language of touch', *Nursing Research*, 28, 2, 76-80.

Wertz, F. (1983), 'Some constituents of descriptive psychological reflection', *Human Studies*, 6, 35-51.

Wertz, F. (1985), 'Method and Findings in a Phenomenological Psychological Study of a Complex Life-Event: Being Criminally Victimized', in Giorgi, A. (ed.), *Phenomenology and Psychological Research*, Duquesne University Press, Pittsburgh.

Wertz, F. (1986), 'The question of the reliability of psychological research', *Journal of Phenomenological Psychology*, 17, 2, 181-205.

Westin, A. (1967), *Privacy and Freedom*, Atheneum, New York.

Willcocks, D.; Peace, S. and Kellaher, L. (1987), *Private Lives in Public Places*, Tavistock Publications, London.

Williams, M. (1988), 'The physical environment and patient care', *Annual Review of Nursing Research*, 6, 3, 61-84.

Williamson, C. (1992), *Whose Standards? Consumer and Professional Standards in Health Care*, Open University Press, Buckingham.

Wilson, H. and Hutchinson, S. (1991), 'Triangulation of qualitative methods: heideggerian hermeneutics and grounded theory', *Qualitative Health Research*, 1, 2, 263-76.

Winogrond, I. (1981), 'A comparison of interpersonal distancing behavior in young and elderly adults', *International Journal of Aging and Human Development*, 13, 1, 53-60.

Wondolowski, C. and Davis, D. (1991), 'The lived experience of health in the oldest old: a phenomenological study', *Nursing Science Quarterly*, 4, 3, 113-8.

Young, J. (1978), 'Introduction: A Look at Privacy', in Young, J. (ed.). *Privacy*, John Wiley and Sons, Chichester.

Younger, K. (1972), *Report of the Committee on Privacy*, Her Majesty's Stationery Office, London.

Youngman, M. (1978), *Designing and Analysing Questionnaires*, TRC, Oxford.

Zimring, C.; Carpman, J. and Michelson, W. (1987), 'Design for Special Populations: Mentally Retarded Persons, Children, Hospital Visitors', in Stokol, D. and Altman, I. (eds), *Handbook of Environmental Psychology, Volume I and II*, John Wiley & Sons, New York.